FAT EQUALS THIN

the hidden power behind being overweight

by

Michael Gers

Published by:

Kima Global Publishers
P.O.Box 374,
RONDEBOSCH
7701
SOUTH AFRICA

Website: **http://www.globalvisions.org/cl/kima**
e-mail: **kima@gem.co.za**

First Edition May 1997

Copyright Michael Gers 1997

ISBN 0-9584065-3-7

World rights Kima Global Publishers. All rights reserved. With the exception of small extracts quoted for review purposes, no part of this publication may be reproduced, translated, adapted, stored in retrieval system, or transmitted in any form or through any means including electronic, mechanical, photocopying, recording or otherwise without the written permission of the publisher.

Cover design: Fiona C.Fisher
Set in 10pt.Century Schoolbook
Printed in South Africa

Contents

	A Few Words	1
One:	Creating Results	7
	Understanding.....the effortless way	10
Two:	The Dance of Energy	15
Three:	Self-empowerment	25

THE MENTAL BODY power of imagination, 28 disconnected images, connected images, the thought loop, creative visualisation, re-framing your thought pictures, the sub-conscious mind, self-affirmations, general affirmations, specific affirmations.

THE EMOTIONAL BODY transmuting emot-59 ion, directing emotion, the thought loop

THE PHYSICAL BODY body awareness exer-69 cise, the power of physiology, the physiology loop

THE SPIRITUAL BODY Higher Self medita- 76 tion, everything serves a purpose

Four:	Beyond Success or Failure	89
	....about restoring balance	93
Five:	The Beauty of Self	105
	SELF-LOVE	106
	SELF-BELIEF The power of collective beliefs, the power of personal beliefs	115
	SELF-RESPONSIBILITY	128
Six:	Power Tools	133
	INSPIRATION	133
	MOTIVATION external motivation, internal motivation	138
	VISION SETTING Your Body Vision, short-term visions, medium-term visions, long-term visions	142
	PRIORITISING	152
	PASSION POWER	155
	THE ESSENCE OF TIME	157
	THE EBB AND FLOW CYCLE	160

	RE-FRAMING	161
	PERSONAL POTENTIAL	165
Seven:	**Eating for Pleasure**	**169**
	"YOU" THE DYNAMIC INDIVIDUAL, the R.D.A. factor, the Diet!	172
	EATING INTUITIVELY When to eat! The denial loop, need or desire, What to eat! How much to eat!	183
Eight:	**A Passing Enjoinder**	**203**

A Few Words....

This book grew out of a need, a need to be able to lose weight without the necessity of having to impose discipline, or deny the pleasure of eating. It was a quest that began more than twenty-five years ago: a journey of self-discovery that was to lead to a deeper understanding of the boundless dimensions of personal potential.

There are two paths to losing weight: that of will-power, the other that of self-empowerment. Will-power requires discipline and self-denial. And, as we all know so well, discipline is only required when we dislike doing something. On the other hand, that which we take pleasure in, does not call for discipline, or denial. Self-empowerment embraces that which comes naturally to one. It does not demand unmitigated effort - nor the imposition of will-power. Self-empowerment is the celebration of gratification and fulfilment.

Fat Equals Thin is a dynamic approach to losing and sustaining weight loss that is based on the principal: *If you have been able to effectively create yourself FAT, then you can effectively create yourself THIN.*

In order to create yourself overweight you need to be empowered. You need to have developed an effective and powerful 'strategy' that engages your ability to mentally visualize, emotionally respond, and physiologically back up your intentions. You cannot create yourself overweight unless you are capable of applying these resources consistently over an extended period of time. Being overweight is testimony to your empowerment.

To lose weight, you need to understand how you shape your thoughts, what emotional responses you infuse to back up your mental imagery, what physiological responses you effect and how you connect with your spiritual essence in order to create yourself overweight. By changing the modalities of your 'strategy' you hold the key to losing weight and re-directing your choices. As you will discover, if you are capable of gaining weight, you have all the resources you need to lose weight - **Fat Equals Thin**.

As long as you are mentally capable of directing your thoughts you have the awesome potential for realizing your dreams and fulfilling your aspirations. Every action and decision that you make comes from the same power source. It is all a matter of how you direct this power.

"People already have the resources they need in order to change if they can be helped to have the appropriate resources in the appropriate context."[1]

Fat Equals Thin embraces the concept of being able to creatively view the behavioral patterns that created you overweight in a new and enabling way. This re-frame empowers you to transform **Fat** into **Thin**. Re-framing literally means placing a larger more expansive frame around an issue; being able to enlarge and change your frame of reference and in so doing change your responses.

---

[1] *Frogs into Princes* - by Grinder and Bandler, Real People Press

Fat Equals Thin is divided into a number of phases. The first of these phases deals with an in-depth understanding of *how you function*: how to access and direct your mental, emotional, physical, and spiritual resources.

The second phase concerns *restoring balance* - understanding what psychological purpose being overweight serves. The sole purpose of overweight, obesity, illness, or any other form of imbalance is to make one whole. The body is the means by which the mind can reveal that which needs attending to.

Overweight or illness are signs that point to that which we have failed to integrate at a conscious level. As hunger is symptomatic of a need, so over-eating is symptomatic of a need to address unresolved past psychological issues and traumas. Over-weight, dis-ease or any other physical imbalance is the body's attempt at re-creating balance. Through the physical manifestation of being overweight the symptom restores balance.

At all levels the holistic body (that is; spirit, mind, emotions, and body) is naturally inclined towards a state of balance. Being overweight is an attempt to regain balance - to restore harmony and alignment. This section reveals how to discover what 'need' being overweight fulfils for you and how to re-create balance without having to overeat.

The third phase deals with the establishment of a set of conditions that supports and aligns you in your quest to lose weight.

The fourth phase presents you with the means to draw on some of your additional resources - your "*power tools*". These tools enable you to give impetus and direction to losing weight.

Finally, the last phase deals with *'eating for pleasure'* - an easy, intuitive approach that embraces the awareness that your nutritional needs are dynamic; that they vary from day to day, moment to moment, and from individual to individual. As you go about your day what you mentally, emotionally, physically, and spiritually experience determines what you need to eat. Sitting on a beach is not quite the same experience as facing a business or personal crisis!

If you eat what you need, not only will you be able to effortlessly lose weight and sustain this weight loss, but you will enjoy health, beauty, and fulfilment.

This section explains how to access your innate intuitive intelligence and how you can lose weight without having to deny the pleasure of eating.

Fat Equals Thin is concerned with teaching you how to simply and effectively re-channel your resources. The ability to direct your empowerment means that you can purposefully direct your life without having to impose discipline, will-power, or effort. Through a deeper understanding of your innate empowerment you can chart an effortless course to weight-loss and self-attainment.

This approach is not only concerned with how to lose weight, but also how to find fulfilment. The ability to give meaning and direction in one area presupposes that you have the same capacity and ability for attainment in any other area of your life. The principals and processes that are involved in losing weight can be applied to all areas of your life. Self-empowerment concerns everything you do or wish to do. You can direct your empowerment to create yourself slim and firm, or you can use these resources to make a million! The choice is yours.

Fat Equals Thin is intended as a hands-on approach to self-attainment. By working through the exercises you ensure that you are not simply acquiring more data about losing weight - you are creating the basis for a deeper understanding of your limitless potentiality. Personal participation is essential to the process of actualizing your dreams and visions. In Buddhism, *tantra* is a sanskrit word that is used to describe the practice of the philosophy. Its meaning is 'to weave' - to merge learning with application. For meaningful change to take place, you have to shift from merely being an observer to becoming a participator. In this process, is the discovery of self-potential and the reward of self-fulfilment.

It can be stated that there is inferred knowledge, and direct knowledge. Inferred knowledge is knowledge that has not been integrated into one's life. Direct knowledge involves the experiencing of that which is known. This is the state of understanding. This is the process of individuation and the road to fulfilment.

It is important to mention at this point that it is not necessary to intellectually assimilate the concepts that are advanced. Rather, it is of far more benefit that you gain a *sense* of the underlying essence of what is being said. Allow that part of your mind that is often referred to as your unconscious mind to assist you in the process of assimilation. The conscious mind is great on installing strategies but not always that effective at running these strategies. Once you have learnt to write, for example, you do not need to use your intellect to put pen to paper, walk, or perform the numerous other functions that you engage in daily. In fact, if you were to mentally intrude in the many actions you perform unconsciously the results would be calamitous. So once you have read through the material and have absorbed what you need to know, relax and allow your innate intelligence to assist you.

Throughout the various chapters you are requested to write down your response to specific situations. It is important that you work through the relevant sections. Articulation necessitates that you be clear about your thoughts. It is a step beyond merely entertaining an assumption. It is a means of focusing and shaping your thoughts, intentions and visions. Through participating in the written exercises you begin the process of enacting the principles and processes contained within the material so that by the time you have finished reading this book, you are already **creating results**.

Chapter One

Creating Results

Dieting represents a multi-billion dollar industry. Statistics reveal that **98% of all dieters fail** - that is they regain all the weight they may have lost, plus interest[2]. The fact that overweight people are still so prevalent in our society is evidence that something essential to the equation of weight loss is missing.

You may start off with the greatest of intentions, but somewhere along the line you waver and give up. You may lose weight for a period of time but achieving a lasting benefit is seldom attained. The discipline and suppression of your desires creates states of conflict and dejection. Your associations of dieting may include self-statements like; "I hate dieting", "I loathe my body", or, "Food is my enemy". What begins as an inspired intention to lose weight often ends with a feeling of futility at ever becoming slim again. Yet, at the same time you have a deep sense that under the right conditions you have the capacity to be thin. This is confirmed by your endless attempts to try yet again!

Consider that if you have effectively put **on** weight that you can effectively **lose** weight. The power of *Fat* is the power of *Thin*.[3] The missing link

---

[2] *Overcoming Eating* by Jane R.Hirschmann and Carol H.Munter published by Cedar.
[3] 'Thin' is a relative concept. It is for you to define a body weight that you are comfortable with and that relates to your natural body weight and unique shape, rather than projecting an idealized

to the equation of being thin is **self-empowerment** - the boundless ability to re-direct your energy in unlimited ways.

We all have the capacity to attain. You may have chosen to develop your career, pursue an interest in sport or some other area of your life - or even create yourself overweight. These are simply choices you exercise. Every decision and action you take, comes from the same power source. It is merely a matter of how you direct your power - what choices you make. Just as the power of water can be devastating in a flood so the same power can be harnessed to provide the benefit of hydro-electricity. As long as you are mentally capable of directing your thoughts you hold the unlimited capacity for directing your life and realizing your aspirations.

I would like you to consider that there is no such thing as failure. Failure is an attitude rather than a consequence. If you view the consequence of your actions as that of having failed, then you have failed. But if you view the consequences of your actions as an opportunity for personal growth and expansion then you have not failed. You have in effect moved forward; and it is only through moving forward that personal growth and self-attainment is possible.

One of my dreams as a teenager was to be able to develop my body. For many years (something like fifteen years) I struggled to develop my physique. No matter how hard I trained, no matter what I did, I just could not seem to achieve the results I wanted.

---

bodyweight and shape that is associated with the likes of models and film stars. 'Thin' should be determined by what it takes to make you feel good about yourself.

Being what is referred to in gym circles as a 'hard gainer' - someone who's genetics are not ideally suited to bodybuilding meant that my body did not respond readily to exercise. In my endeavour to beat my genetic limitations I was obliged not only to experiment with different physical and nutritional approaches but I was also induced to explore many different areas and fields of study. I was prodded into being twice as smart in order to make gains. I read and researched everything I could get my hands on. Each apparent 'failure' broadened and enhanced my knowledge and understanding. Each 'failure' provided me with the insight and opportunity for personal growth and discovery. I often wonder whether I would be writing this book now if I had not 'failed' so successfully. So in my case my gift as a teenager was my shapeless body!

Belief in failure imposes a limitation on your ability to make choices. If you regard the outcome of any situation as part of your growth and future success then you have not failed. Each outcome places you closer to achieving your goal. The process can be likened to that of a plane's navigator who is continually forced to re-adjust for strong winds and air currents to reach the intended destination. It is virtually impossible for a plane to fly in a straight line from point A, to point B. The navigator "tacks" from one point to another until the plane finally reaches its destination. This process of "tacking" is a learning process, a process that enables you to keep on fine-tuning your approach as you continually discover new and exciting potentials. This is a process of self-enrichment. Once you have set an intention and initiate the process of moving forward there will be times where it will appear that you are meandering off course. These are your growth points. If you no longer view these outcomes as either good or bad, negative or positive, but see that the outcome of any action as merely a result, then you are no longer disempowered. You are now in a position to make choices that were not previously available.

Fat Equals Thin is a dynamic approach that will enable you to re-direct your empowerment to becoming slim and healthy. There is no actual impediment that can prevent you from losing weight other than the way in which you view yourself.

We are all endowed with extraordinary attributes; the mind, emotions, body and spirit are capable of unlimited and extraordinary potentialities. You need only to reflect on your ability to imagine, to dream, to have a vision of what you want - to begin to sense the magnitude of your empowerment; for within your dreams and visions are contained the seeds of attainment.

Losing weight should not merely be viewed as an end result. It should rather be seen as a process. It is a means of discovering things about yourself that you would otherwise have avoided looking at. By facing these issues you attain the ability to control your weight and acquire the understanding and strength to succeed in other areas of your life. The essence of your power lies within. **You** are the source.

Through a deeper understanding of yourself you can chart an effortless course to self-attainment.

Understanding.... the Effortless Way

We live in an age of ever increasing knowledge and information. As such we have become the receptors of a deluge of data. At times it seems impossible to keep abreast of this tidal wave of knowledge and information. Yet, when we look around us there appears to be little evidence of any commensurate advance in personal fulfilment. Social and personal distress is exponentially on the increase.

What then is the value of all this information? Surely we must conclude that knowledge in itself does not adequately fulfil our personal needs. The question must also be asked: Why is it that knowledge that concerns human development is not being integrated into people's lives? What is missing? It is obvious that it is simply not enough to know about dieting or any other area related to personal development. What is needed is the ability to be able to enact this knowledge - to put this knowledge into practice.

At this stage it is important that we examine the difference between that which is defined as **knowledge**, and that which is defined as **understanding**. Knowledge refers to cognition; it is the apprehension of information. For example, you can assume that as a result of losing weight that your health and energy levels will improve. In addition you may benefit from a lowering of your cholestrol levels. This knowledge enables you to make an informed assessment of the situation. But the knowledge of all this does not necessarily mean that you will be able to effect this knowledge and change your attitudes and responses.

No amount of knowledge is going to propel you into action if you are not *'moved'* to bring about change. I say *'moved'* because there is another vital ingredient that is necessary before you effect knowledge and bring about personal change.

When it comes to losing weight there is no shortage of dietary knowledge that promises the miraculous. Many of these dietary approaches, aside from the fads, may in essence be nutritionally correct and balanced in their approach and yet it appears that we are still unable to effortlessly and permanently lose weight.

The difference between a temporary and a lasting state of weight loss can be defined as the difference between knowledge and understanding. *Understanding* is a state of being that enables one to effortlessly enact *knowledge*. It is a stage beyond knowledge - beyond the activities of the conscious mind. Until knowledge is infused with the breath of *understanding*, it remains dormant.

Understanding refers to synchronous comprehension, a simultaneous 'whole' knowing, an awareness that involves your mental, emotional, physical, and spiritual being. It is a deep complete realization - a state of understanding that brings with it an actual shift - a movement - a revelation! Understanding transfers knowledge into action without effort. There is no separation between what you think, and what you feel - you simply enact. If you look back on your life you will be able to identify situations when you 'saw' something with such clarity that you were able to enact change there and then. This experience, this deep realization propelled you into action. You were not divided as to whether to do, or not to do. You did not equivocate. You did not change your mind three days later, three months later, or even three years later.

On the other hand you have experienced situations where you have decided to do something only to waver and give up. For example, you may have decided to give up smoking, go to gym every morning, or lose weight. Somehow, somewhere along the line you lose your resolve and give up. This inability to see something through to completion can be attributed to the lack of synchronous comprehension - to a lack of understanding. In other words, if you set an intention and did not see it through, you made a 'partial' decision. You made a decision based on only one of your centres. You possibly made a mental decision to lose weight, or you made a decision based on an emotional response; but whatever you did, you did not make a combined decision involving all your centres. You were not 'moved' to bring about change. As a result of making a partial decision, you created internal conflict. Your head was saying one thing, your emotions another, and your body and spirit something else. Once you have internal conflict there is only one way that you can direct change and that is through the imposition of will-power and discipline, the constraints of which demand unmitigated effort. And, as we all know so well, anything that demands discipline and effort is invariably doomed to fail.

Understanding the need to lose weight means that you need to mentally perceive, emotionally feel, physically sense, and spiritually be aware of the need to enact change. Once all these parts form the whole, you have a collective energy and understanding that moves you to effortlessly transform weight gain into weight loss. It is essential that you therefore become aware of your various bodies and develop a deeper awareness of their integrated and potential functions.

Understanding bridges the gap between knowledge and enaction, imbalance and balance, the part and the whole. Through the harmonious alignment of all your bodies (mental, physical, emotional and spiritual), a powerful and effortless transformation takes place. This is the enabling state of self empowerment and the underlying intent of ***Fat Equals Thin***.

But, before dealing with the various expressions that constitute the fullness of empowerment, it is necessary to grasp the notion that there is an enabling way of viewing human potential that is not bounded by what you may have been taught to believe.

Chapter Two

The Dance of Energy

"There are many signs that the next great adventure for humanity will take place in the realm of consciousness, and that a whole range of unexplored possibilities awaits us.

In the new view of human life which is just emerging, man's inner resources are seen to embody not only his physical systems but also a process for replenishing vitality, and an almost untapped resource of higher energies which can harmonize and integrate the mind and emotions with the physical body, thus enhancing all of life."[4]

There is an arising awareness that life as we experience it through our senses can no longer simply be attributed to the consequence of chemical and physical processes. Beyond the organizational patterning of the RNA/DNA molecule and the sub-atomic realm of particles, a renewed vista is emerging. Where our modern perspective has been coloured by science and chemistry, our future panorama of human potential is once again being shaped by an awareness that energy is the basis to all of life. Once again, in that it seems that we are completing a sequence. A sequence that much like the spiralling orbit of the hundred billion galaxies

---

[4] *The Chakras and the Human Energy Fields* by Shafica Karagulla M.D., and Dora van Gelder-Kunz, a Quest book, The Theosophical Publishing House.

that make up our universe, eventually completes a cycle and begins anew.

This sequence, this history, of man's inner development began with the worship of the presence and power of nature: the force of the frozen glacial shifts that etched their primordial shapes into the mantle of the earth, the violent flaring of volcanoes that spewed their molten lava from the bowels of the earth, the wild fury of thunderbolts flaring across darkened skies, the rejuvenation of the seasons, the celebration of birth; in all these things early man sensed the connectedness of nature and the creative power of energy.

As we now round the bend of this century and come to the end of another millennium there is no doubt that we are poised on the edge of sweeping change, not only technologically and socially, but also personally. Our systems of thought are undergoing a necessary and expansive transformation.

In our quest for personal advancement it is imperative that we once again take cognizance of the recognition that a dynamic energetic intelligence constitutes the backcloth to all of life. The issue of viewing ourselves in terms of dynamic energy rather than immutable physical matter is an enabling approach for it allows us to be the beneficiaries of a restorative endowment - *to create without limitation.*

Beneath the surface of what we perceive as the physical or material world, lies yet another 'reality',......a reality not fixed by any concept of the separation of mind and matter, but rather a reality enchanted by a magic that permeates all of life. In his book *The Secret of the Creative Vacuum*, John Davidson describes this condition, "..........*So this matrix is around and surrounding us, if we can but tune in to its scintillating, vibrant, natural, awesome, yet delicate symphony."* The words 'tune in', suggest an approach that is of a subtle nature rather than that of unmitigated effort. It is also a suggestion that the laws of the universe follow the laws of harmonic resonance rather than that of mechanistic principles.

As dynamic, energetic beings we are like tuning forks: when a tuning fork is struck it causes a sympathetic resonance and corresponding sound in other tuning forks of the same key. In ancient Greece aeolian harps were mounted on the ragged cliffs of the Aeolian islands. These wind harps were attuned and conceived to resound to the fluctuation of the wind. The gentle breezes sweeping along the shoreline created delicate harmonies quite different to the dissenting discordance of storm driven winds. The angle of deflection, the velocity, each subtle aspect of the wind determined the music that was created. Each melody was unique. In effect we are no different: we are also like aeolian harps reverberating to energy frequencies. We are delicately attuned to resonate with all of life.

If we develop this suggestion that we are composed of dynamic energy fields then a whole new world of creativity is opened up to us. We speak of something striking 'a lost chord' in us or of being 'in tune'. In a way this is a recognition that we are composed of dynamic energy even if we are not aware of the significance of what we are saying. Being receptive to energy imparts valuable information about ourselves and the situations that affect us. It aids our development. As we unfold and develop this sensitivity and awareness we increase our ability to create effortlessly.

The world we live in is a world of energy. The essence to all of matter, whether it be animate or inanimate, is that of vibrating energy. Every creative impulse and every expression is a response to energy. Sensitives that are able to read the body's energy fields describe bands of glowing colours that emanate from the body.[5]

The ability to respond to energy is not a faculty that is limited to psychics, or clairvoyants. If you have ever sensed the beauty and presence of a forest or cathedral then you have sensed energy. If you have ever referred to someone as giving off bad 'vibes' then you have sensed energy. Momentarily reflect on your daily life and you will begin to realize that you rely on your intuitive responses to energy a great deal more than what you may be inclined to acknowledge. When you consider the act of eating and how the body functions you are considering energy. If you talk about losing weight or putting on weight you are talking about energy. The heady experience of being in love is the experience of energy. Every situation concerns the exchange of energy. We live in world of pulsating energy. We are energy beings.

So, whether you talk of thoughts, feelings, losing weight, a supernova giving birth to a cluster of planets or spiritual awareness you are essentially talking about the manifestation of energy.

The concept of energy is not a new one. Since the dawning of mankind, different cultures, religions, and spiritual teachings have detailed and made mention of human energy fields: Taoism, Buddhism,

---

[5] As a form of vibratory energy, colour has a natural capacity to reflect the delicacy and intensity of thoughts and emotions.

Sufism, Jewish mysticism, the ancient Vedic texts of Hinduism, to name but a few. The Milesians of ancient Greece were referred to as "hylozoists" or "those that think matter is alive"[6]. The Milesians did not differentiate between animate and inanimate or body and soul. They fostered a world view of unified organic life energy. Other ancient Greek writings also make mention of vital energies: Hippocrates makes reference to a fluid-like energy that flowed through the body. Chinese Taoism of the 3rd millennium BCE[7] describes energy as 'chi', or the 'breath' that binds mind, body and spirit together to form a connection between our inner and outer worlds. At a symbolic level there are many examples of Christian reference to spiritual energy. Pictorial and sculptural representations of Christ and other religious figures are depicted with mandalas of light surrounding their crown areas. Energy, however it is described, pervades every level of our existence whether we choose to be aware of it or not!

One of our problems with trying to grasp the notion of a world linked together by dynamic webs of energy can largely be attributed to Western science's description of the physical world and how these ideas have impacted on our view of ourselves. For nearly three hundred years Newtonian physics has held sway over our perception of nature. Newtonian physics holds that the fundamental building blocks of nature are comprised of atoms: a nucleus of protons and neutrons with electrons orbiting around the nucleus. This concept of the very quintessence of

---

[6] *The Tao of Physics* by Fritjof Capra published by Flamingo
[7] BCE/CE Before Common Era/Common Era, a more universal and less judgmental convention than BC/AD.

nature embodies the notion that atoms are made up of immutable solid parts, rather than particles of resonating energy. This view is the summation of a line of thought that began in the 6th century BCE in Greece. The Eleatic school held that mind and matter were separate. Matter was regarded as being essentially comprised of inactive atoms that depended on their movement from some outside divine source. This dualistic concept of mind (consciousness) and matter, with matter being comprised of immutable solid particles that were incapable of being influenced by the mind, continued to find expression through to the 17th century CE, where it reached its apogee in the Cartesian philosophy of René Descartes and the mechanistic physics of Newton.

Newtonian mechanics was able to successfully predict the motions of the sun, moon and planets, mechanical machines and all those every day matters that touch our lives - like why falling apples eventually come to rest. The material world was viewed as though it were a huge machine. So successful was this mechanistic model of Newtonian thought that we are still inclined to experience our bodies in a mechanical way and think of ourselves as being composed of 'solid' matter, rather than as dynamic patterns of energy.

As much as our past is steeped in Newtonian mechanics, supported by the pillars of Cartesian thought, our future is sallying headlong into an enigmatic world where even quantum physics is now proclaiming the connectedness of all of life.[8] Where

---

[8] For an accessible explanation read *Activation for Ascension* by David Ash, published by Kima Global Publishers.

once the forces and laws of gravity painted a picture of an ordered, predictable cosmos, the forces of quantum physics are now suggesting an enfolded order suffused and connected by mutable energy.

"......According to particle physics, the world is fundamentally dancing energy; energy that is everywhere and incessantly assuming first this form and then that. What we have been calling matter (particles) constantly is being created, annihilated and created again......Physicists found themselves dealing with energy that somehow processed information (which made it organic), and unaccountably presented itself in patterns (waves). In short, physicists found themselves dealing with Wu Li - patterns of organic energy.[9]

Not only does quantum physics recognize that the basis to all matter is vibrant energy it also acknowledges the importance of the observer in determining the outcome of the experiment. Quantum physics tells us that the observer/ mind/ consciousness influences the consequence of what is experienced. Between setting up and measuring the outcome of an experiment, the observer becomes an integral part of the whole process. The *interaction* of the observer determines what is experienced. Just as the physicist Arthur Compton proved that light is able to exert a pressure and influence matter, so too consciousness is capable of influencing what we experience.

Newtonian science held that it was not necessary to include the observer in its model of the

---

[9] *The Dancing Wu Li Masters* by Gary Zukav, Rider, an imprint of Random Century Group Ltd.

universe. It was felt that the universe could be explained objectively without the presence of man. The integration of the observer (consciousness) is an imperative move towards the recognition that both man and the universe are linked in some integral way.

In 1935 two researchers, Dr. Harold Saxton Burr and Dr. F. Northrop of Yale managed to show that all forms of life have energy fields and that these electro-magnetic fields, or L-fields as they were called are *".....the organizational 'mechanisms' that keep the physical life form in shape and carry out maintenance and repair through the constant inflow of new material"*[10] In association with leading researchers in many other medical fields Dr. Burr was able to demonstrate a relationship between health and L-fields. Dr Burr extended his experiments over a wide range of areas. He was also able to detect that the L-fields of trees fluctuated according to the phases of the moon, sunspots, and magnetic storms.

In addition to the work done by Dr. Burr and many others in this field of research the advent of technologies like the X-ray, CAT scanners and laser technology has furnished further evidence of the existence of human energy fields. I am sure that at some time or another you have had an X-ray, or a scan. These procedures would not have been possible if you were not comprised of dynamic energy fields.

The recognition of vital energy fields offers us the opportunity of new, broader vistas to personal potential and well-being. The capacity for energy to transmute one state into another - whether it be

---

[10] *Blueprint for Immortality* by Dr.Harold Saxton Burr published by C.W.Daniel

water into steam, or weight gain into weight loss, is an enabling potential for replenishing vitality, restoring health and re-creating balance. This endowment is revealed in the natural law that states: *energy follows thought.* This axiom is an enabling paradigm for it pronounces the connective link between what you think and what you manifest.

What you think - the way in which you direct your energy is vital to the process of losing weight and sustaining health.

So, finally it seems that we are arriving at a point where confirmation of the observations made by the ancients as they gazed out in awe at the celestial bodies and payed homage to the changing seasons from their stone temples and hilltops is being reconfirmed mathematically and experimentally in the sanctums of technology and science. From the tracks of sub-atomic particles etched on photographic plates in bubble-chambers, and implications of superluminal transfer of information, a holographic image of the universe is emerging - a universe where mind and matter are inextricably linked together by the vivifying dance of energy. This dance of energy reaches beyond the conceptual confines of solid immutable matter: for a proton is no longer simply a proton, nor is a neutron simply a neutron.

The dance of energy unfolds in a pirouette that is as fascinating as it is astounding. The implications of this extends beyond mere science; for we are now caught up in a dance where the extremities of physics and metaphysics are beginning to stir to the same consonance. Each swirl of the dance proclaims the connection between creation and energy. Each step takes us closer to the point where it is possible to create without effort or limitation. Each stride celebrates the *power of self*.

CHAPTER 3

Self-Empowerment

Self-empowerment is the realization of 'all' that you are: it is the fundamental recognition that your limitless power and beauty comes from within, not from without. This is not something that has to be acquired or learnt for it has always been there and always will be there. The only thing that separates you from being empowered - from losing weight, or achieving in any other area of your life, is the way in which you view yourself - the separation between *what you are,* and *what you think you are.*

As we develop from childhood through adolescence and then on to adulthood we decide on the basis of past experiences what is possible, and what is impossible. These beliefs determine our potential - they colour our perception of ourselves. One of our greatest misconceptions is that we think that the road to self-attainment or weight loss is an arduous and energy consuming process. Contained within this are the beliefs; 'nothing comes easy', 'no pain, no gain'. Nothing can be further from the truth. These beliefs are not universal truths. As you will begin to discover, it is not a matter of developing your ability to achieve but rather releasing that which stands in the way of self-attainment. By re-framing the beliefs and concepts that restrict your ability to attain you are initiated into a realm that knows no bounds.

There are no limitations to your personal potential. The fact that you may not have lost weight effortlessly in the past, firewalked, seen auras, written a best-selling novel or made a million dollars does not mean that you are incapable of these acts. Much of what we believe about ourselves is limited by what we have experienced in the past. It is important to understand that *just as you are not your thoughts, so you are not your experiences.* No surgeon will ever be able to find your past experiences lodged in your brain, or any other part of your anatomy for that matter. Those past experiences that limit your ability to attain only have power when you claim them, that is, when you believe they are a part of you.

You are whole and complete as you are. You enact as a 'whole' being. Everything you do, whether it be eating, walking, falling in love or any other activity is based on being whole. These acts are the consequences of your thoughts, feelings, physical responses and spiritual connection. There is nothing that you do that is not the result of the simultaneous interaction of your holistic body. You do not simply think a thought and then act out your intention without involving your mental, emotional, physical and spiritual bodies.

Certain actions and situations may seem to involve more of one expression than of another. Solving a mathematical problem will certainly involve more of your mental expression than your spiritual expression. On the other hand facing a moral issue will appear to concern mostly emotional and spiritual expression. But, whatever you do simultaneously involves all four bodies. Your bodies are connected - they touch each other and are interwoven to form a tapestry of extraordinary balance, beauty and potential. What affects one body affects all your other bodies.

The fact that you are not normally aware of this fusion, this connectedness between your four bodies, in no way invalidates the functioning of these bodies. The functioning of one's senses is a good analogy of how this principle operates. Normally one is aware only of two or three senses. For example when you eat, you may only be aware of your senses of taste, sight and smell, yet be unaware of the functioning of your auditory and feeling senses. These seemingly excluded senses continue to function and are inextricably involved in the process of eating, even though you may not be conscious of the information that is being put out by these 'neglected' senses. The inclusion of these senses only requires that you expand the focus of your awareness - that you become fully attentive to the information that is being given to you. Similarly, the inclusion of all your four bodies requires only that you begin to expand your awareness. Whatever you do, whether it be eating, composing a melody, or simply making a cup of tea involves the consequence of your mental, emotional, physical, and spiritual actions.

The wisdom and empowerment of your holistic body is always available. The recognition that you have available the combined intelligence and energy of your holistic body increases your power to attain weight loss and self-fulfilment. As you expand and develop your awareness of the connectedness of all your bodies this awareness re-aligns your various bodies releasing the combined energy and power of all your 'parts' - the sum of which is greater than the parts. This holistic power is the key to effortless attainment and enduring weight loss.

Paradoxically though, it is through understanding each part, each body separately, that we are able to comprehend the whole. Comprehension can be compared to listening to a symphony - you need to listen to each movement separately in order to be able to experience the whole. The parts that form your holistic body are; your mental, emotional, physical and spiritual bodies. The fact that they are dealt with separately does not in any way imply that they function separately. As Danah Zohar states *".... their 'individual' existences derive both their definition and their meaning from that whole"*[1]

The Mental Body

"With the power of your mind you can create whatever you wish. It is you and you alone, that forms the nature of the world in which you live."[2]

If you are unable to direct your thoughts, you are unable to direct your life. Its as simple as that! Any decision that you make, any behaviour you effect, any action you take, is all a response to thought.

Just as your body reflects the external world so your mind reflects your inner world.

The world of thought originates in the mind which is linked to the body through the brain. In turn the brain derives information from the external world by means of the senses. The mind uses the brain to realise its intentions. And, this is where we come to a rather subtle distinction; the mind is not to be found in the brain, or for that matter anywhere else in the physical body. For the mind is in the words of Paul Davies, *"... a tenuous, elusive, ethereal sort of substance, the stuff that thoughts and dreams are made of"*[3]

---

[1] *The Quantum Self* by Danah Zohar published by Flamingo
[2] *The Vision of Ramala* published by C.W.Daniel
[3] *God and the New Physics* by Paul Davies published by Penguin.

As the mind is not of the brain, but rather a pervasive state of being, it is necessary to become aware that thoughts are not governed by some uncontrollable outside force. Thoughts are determined by the act of free-will. What you think, how you direct your thoughts, are a choice you make, moment to moment.

When it comes to enacting change there are basically two ways in which thought can be directed: 'Creative visualization' - the way in which you consciously use powerful visual images and 'Reframing' - modifying the way in which you mentally 'represent' thoughts.

These choices, whether they be in response to thoughts that are generated by the senses (from the outside in), or, whether they be thoughts that generate physical activity (from the inside out), are all determined by how you choose to respond. This focus of choice implies that you can choose to be fat, or you can choose to be thin.

Thoughts are merely frequencies of energy. If you think negatively you generate negative energy frequencies and accordingly act negatively. The more you begin to realize this inalienable relationship between the thoughts you think and the actions you take the more you will come to acknowledge that you have the power to create and the prerogative of choice. The fact that you have created yourself overweight is proof that you are empowered. If you have effectively put on weight, then you can effectively lose weight - **Fat Equals Thin**. Thoughts are self-determined, they are not imposed on you by someone else or by anything else for that matter.

Thought is dynamic - not only is it capable of being directed, but it has the ability to stretch beyond the limitations of the physical world. Through thought, through imagination, you hold the power to create.

The Power of Imagination

One of the most startling revelations about the brain is its inability to discern the difference between that which is perceived to be 'real' and that which is 'imagined'. If I now asked you to sit back and vividly imagine your body as being firm and lean your brain would respond as if the information it was receiving was actual. It would unequivocally believe that your body was indeed slim and firm. In other words, it would not be able to differentiate between imagination, or reality! The implications of this are staggering, for in terms of personal potential the suggestion is one of an expansive capacity to create.

This revelatory fact is not simply conjecture but is based on a large body of scientific research. In his seminal research in the 1930's Edmund Jacobsen discovered that *"... the basal parts of the brain and the central nervous system could not differentiate between something that was actually happening versus something that was being very vividly visualized."*[4]

Another, Maxwell Maltz states *"....the brain and/or nervous system cannot distinguish between an experience that is real and one that is imagined. In other words, an imaginary experience is just as effective in programming attitudes, responses and habits as a real experience. Therefore, any individual can condition himself to success or failure responses by using his imagination to create such responses"*[5]

Imagination is the ability to create mental images. This mental faculty enables you to visualize what you

---

[4] *Mind Power* by Edmund Jacobsen published by Leisure Press.
[5] *Psycho-Cybernetics* by Maxwell Maltz published by Simon and Schuster.

want in the future and is tied to your visions and dreams. Imagination enables you to transcend the limitations of what you believe to be possible. The power of imagination is virtually limitless. Imagination can be said to be the source of conception. For, before you are able to conceive of something you need to be able to hold an image of that which you wish to create in your mind; you need to be able to imagine the act, the circumstance, the end result. You need to be able to unfurl the diverse possibilities of your intention. This applies to all areas, whether you are involved in creating yourself slim, painting a picture, or solving a mathematical problem.

Imagination is the bough of potentiality - a connective link that branches outward in its reach for expansiveness. It is rooted in the mind's inclination for boundless attainment.

The great thinkers of all ages have relied on imagination for their most creative work. Einstein, one of the greatest minds of all time, acknowledged that there was an important link between abstract science and imagination. Yet, another distinguished physicist, Max Plank, had this to say about being a formative scientist; *"... a vivid intuitive imagination for new ideas not generated by deduction, but by artistically creative imagination."*

Whether you are aware of it or not you use imagery every day of your life. You use your imagination to arouse your appetite for food. You use imagination to handle situations not yet realized whether this be envisaging how you are going to look once you lose weight, or imagining yourself with a new hairstyle. Imagination helps you to discover what you want. It allows you to test and fine-tune your feelings and responses long before these situations are realized. It is interesting to note that in a study conducted of 500 people, everyone recounted having images of some sort. The statistics reveal that 97% of the group reported visual images.[6] Imagination is part of your potential. The scope of this formative and creative faculty is unbounded.

It is no mere coincidence of nature that one of the fundamental biological functions of the brain is so designed as to facilitate imaginative and creative thought. Since Dr Sperry's breakthrough in the division of left and right brain hemispheres we are now able to recognize the different functions of each side of the brain.[7] Simply put, the left side is responsible for thinking in words and logic. It has the capacity to analyze and separate. The right side thinks in sensory images - in patterns. This side functions more in the non-verbal areas that we have a feeling for. It is our right brain hemisphere that is our source of imagination, creativity, and intuition, and it is our right side which has the capacity for seeing whole patterns, rather than separate aspects.

To gain some idea of the aptitude and power of the brain visualize your brain as having 200,000 times the capacity of the largest computer ever built with 10 billion storage cells. The capacity and potential of the brain can only be described as awesome. Science has suggested that we use only a small percentage of this potential (less than 1%) yet even this is dazzling in its achievements. Through the brain the mind is able to realize its intentions. One of the most effective and creative ways that the mind is able to do this is through imagination.

---

[6] *The Investigation of Mental Images* by P.McKellar Penguin Science Survey.
[7] Even though the two hemispheres perform different functions, they are connected by neural connections. These neural connections ensure complementarity.

Imagination is the process of using images. These images can be described as either 'dis-connected' or 'connected' images. It is important to understand the differences between the two forms of imagery for what we are concerned with, is not only the ability to understand how *you* create your thought pictures, but how you can use your thought pictures to lose weight and direct your empowerment.

Disconnected Images

Disconnected imagery is when you mentally take time out - when you intentionally shift your attention away from what you are doing to something else. Usually this takes the form of visualizing a situation that creates a sense of distraction. You may for example at the end of a demanding exercise regimen or taxing mental problem imagine having a massage. In other words, you disconnect from what you are doing. Disconnected imagery, although a distraction, can be used to mentally refresh and energize yourself. You mentally take time out from stressful situations to imagine something that you find enjoyable or relaxing: you deliberately let your mind wander. I am sure if I asked you to imagine a recent enjoyable experience you would have no problem doing this! The important distinction to be made is that there is a difference between 'daydreaming' and guided mental imagery. Letting your mind wander with intent implies that you are directing your thoughts. When you use 'disconnected' images it is as though you are the projector and you are watching a movie of yourself. One of the forms of this type of imagery is what Jack Schwartz calls the state of 'reverie'. In his book "Voluntary Controls - Exercises for Meditation" he says; "*A reverie can put us in touch with our imaginations and can concentrate our psychic energies and draw them from distractions."* On the other hand when you experience your mental imagery as though it was actually happening to you now, you actually live the experience; you feel, smell, hear and experience the event. In other words you are connected!

Connected Images

Connected imagery is when you are directly connected to what you are imagining. If while exercising you mentally focus on the specific muscles you are working on and simultaneously imagine your body responding to your input then this is connected imagery, or what is otherwise called *'creative visualization'*. Creative visualization can be used in a deeply relaxed state or while involved in some form of activity. Whenever you creatively visualize you are channelling your creative energy to expand and speed up the results.

Creative visualization can used for creating your ideal body, healing, achieving at work, or attaining in any other area of your life. The great thing about creative visualization is that it can be done without effort, and wherever you are. As you go about your day you can feed your body images that endorse your choice to be slim. You can send your body powerful messages of what you want. You can creatively visualize while sitting on the bus, in a waiting room, while cycling on your exercise cycle, meditating, or in any other situation that lends itself to this process. As you begin to integrate visualization into your life you will confirm your creative power by the results you produce. You will validate that *"...you are the constant creator of your life. That is the ultimate point of creative visualization - to make every moment of our lives a moment of wondrous creation, in which we are just naturally choosing the best, the most beautiful, the most fulfilling lives we can imagine "*[8]

When you clearly visualize yourself having lost weight your body enacts this belief. Creative visualization is the ability to consciously direct your imagination. It is a means of using imagination to create what you want in your life by tapping into your creative energy.

Fat Equals Thin

If you created yourself overweight, then you must have used your ability to creatively visualize. There is no way that you can successfully have created yourself overweight, if you were not able to effectively use this faculty. What is now required to create yourself thin, is to make different choices, to re-direct your empowerment - to re-direct your choice of images.

Creative visualization functions at a much deeper level than just 'positive thinking'. Both your conscious and subconscious mind register the image you have visualized and begin to focus the energies necessary for manifestation.

The implication of this is that creative visualization creates an actual neuromuscular response in your body. Your body enacts what you are thinking, even though you may not actually be doing anything. Therefore when you 'think thin', you are programming your body to be slim. By focusing clearly on an image of your body being slim you create the electrical field of a slim body. Quantum physics tells us that where an

---

[8] *Creative Visualization* by Shakti Gawain published by New Age Bantam Books.

electrical field occurs a magnetic field also occurs. We literally draw to ourselves, or magnetize what we think. Dr Karl Pribram an eminent brain researcher from Sybervision advances that through visualization we physically create "...*the specific electro-magnetic properties of that thing."*

Visualization is something you do constantly, whether you are aware of it or not. Whatever you do as you go about your daily activities you are imagining the outcome of your actions, you are visualizing. 'Creative' visualization is a process that creates the blueprint for what you want to achieve. Creative visualization is not something that is just limited to the arts. Even in the disciplines of science and mathematics, creative breakthroughs are the result of imagination and intuition. Whether it be losing weight, playing sport, achieving in business, the arts, relationships, or any other area of your life, in order to achieve you need to consciously use the power of creative visualization. The power of thought is unlimited. In essence, creative visualization is the simple process of focusing on an idea or image in your mind. The more focused and sustained the visual image, the more immediate and effective the manifestation.

It is important that you begin to realize that you are continually creating results. Every thought that goes out into the world is responded to - *energy follows thought*. What you are is the cumulative result of all your previous thoughts. It is not your errant body that caused you to be overweight, it is your collective thoughts and resultant actions that created you overweight. Through your belief systems you create what you are. You are the architect of your body. By choosing to think thin, you are creating a thin blueprint.

Your psyche is continually sending out messages to your body. So if you are fat you have consistently sent out fat messages in the past; and if you now choose to lose weight you need to consistently send out thin messages. The body is unable to discern, it responds literally to the messages it receives.

Thoughts determine what you manifest, they shape your world. Every thought you think is responded to. The greater your focus, the greater your results. By directing your thoughts you have the power to manifest a higher consciousness and open up a world of unlimited possibilities.

The Thought Loop!

Remember that thoughts evoke feelings, and feelings govern your responses. In turn your responses determine your results. So your thoughts ultimately determine your actions and your actions determine what you receive.

Creative Expansion Exercise

This is an exercise that you should do on a regular basis. It requires only a few minutes every day, or, if you can't find the time, at least once a week. It is designed to stimulate your imagination and improve your ability to creatively visualize.

Put down any ideas about what you want in the future. Let yourself go on this one. Do not limit yourself; whatever ideas, dreams or wishes you have, write them down. They don't necessarily have to be related to losing weight or changing your eating patterns. Be expansive and feel the pleasure these things will bring you. This exercise is intended to stimulate your ability to imagine and visualize. Through doing work on the inner plane you are ensuring that your energy is directing what happens on the outer plane. One of the direct benefits of this is that it will save you a lot of unnecessary physical effort in attaining your intention.

....
....
....
....
....
....
....

Creative Visualisation Technique

Creative visualizing can be used to attain any vision on any level; mental, emotional, spiritual, or physical. You can use visualization to create your ideal figure or fill your life with radiance and well-being. Through using powerful expansive images you accelerate your ability to receive in any area of your life.

The first step to creative visualization is being able to relax.[9] The deeper the relaxation, the greater

---

[9] As mentioned previously, creative visualization can also be performed while actively engaged in activity. In this case you would focus on being 'centred' as opposed to being 'relaxed'.

the benefit. Relaxing enables you to slow down your brain-wave patterns, making you responsive to heightened awareness. These slow brain-waves, or alpha waves as they are sometimes referred to, differ from the more active beta waves of the waking state. Researchers have discovered that if you visualize in the alpha state, you are able to effect far greater changes than when you are in a mentally active beta state.

Find a quiet spot. We all have our 'power spots' where we feel particularly comfortable and energized. You should be able to relax and focus your mind without being disturbed either by your family, or the telephone. Those of you that have meditated before will have already established your own approach to relaxing.

Sit, or lie in a comfortable position. Close your eyes and become aware of yourself...... Listen to the sounds, both those outside and inside of you .... Allow these sounds to pass through you.... Now become aware of your sense of smell..... Taste how your mouth feels...... Feel yourself becoming more centred.....Take a few deep breaths and as you exhale, imagine all your tension and worries leaving you.....Watch your breathing, feel its natural rhythm. Now starting with the top of your head, work downward. Feel your face muscles beginning to relax.... Move down your neck and shoulders, feeling the tension draining away ......If you are distracted by thoughts or sounds, merely acknowledge their presence and continue. Move your attention through each part of your body.....down your thighs, knees, calves, ankles, feet and toes ...... Enjoy the feeling of being relaxed.

Relaxation promotes awareness and energy. What you have just practised is a guideline; there are many methods of relaxation. Find what works best for you. The more you practice, the less time it will take for you to become centred.

The next step in the process is to clearly visualize what it is you want; in this case - how you want your figure to look once you have lost weight. When you visualize, visualize something that is possible to create. It may not be realistic to imagine yourself looking like Cindy Crawford, or Claudia Schiffer. Visualize what you believe is possible to create. Once you start experiencing the results you will be able to go onto far bigger things. It is also important that you do not focus on what you **do not want**. Visualization is an *affirmative* process. How you create your images and how you communicate with yourself determines what you will attain. There's a big difference between affirmatively saying to yourself; "I am losing weight", as opposed to the ambiguous self-statement, "I hope I don't put on weight". The only way your body can experience this type of statement is by putting on weight! Be clear about what you want and positively affirm this.. **Do not visualize what you do not want**. How you visualize yourself, determines what you will attain. If you focus on negative images, you will draw these images to you. So, remember, focus on the positive and enabling aspects of what you desire.

Experiment with visualizing; discover what works best for you. It is interesting to note that research has shown that most people visualize an image approximately 20 centimetres in front of their eyes. If this is how you see your images it is important to make this visualization even more a part of yourself by energizing it with a strong feeling of what you want. If when you visualize you do not see a clear picture, there is no need to worry. As you practice creative visualization you will find that with each attempt it will become easier and easier to call up images.

Once you have created your visualization of how you want to look when you have lost weight, place yourself in a setting where people can admire and acknowledge you. You may picture yourself on the beach, wearing a two-piece costume. Imagine yourself as clearly as possible. See the shape of your legs, feel their firmness as you walk past other bathers. Picture the flatness of your stomach and feel the confidence you are exuding. Sense peoples admiration for the way you look. Feel the well-being and beauty you are exuding. Now make the picture clearer.

Make the picture as real as you can; use all your senses to heighten your experience..... Play with enlarging the image of yourself; heighten the colours, sounds and feelings....Envisage wearing the energy of what you will be attracting. Appreciate how this will benefit your life. Learn to integrate your new body before you have it. Whatever qualities you think being slim will give you - beauty, confidence, health, acceptance, - these are the qualities you need to develop. It is these qualities that will make you more magnetic to losing weight. The more inspired you are, the stronger your emotions and feelings will be. Feelings and emotions give enormous power to your mental imagery. In order for visualization to be more than mental concentration, it needs to be energized - it needs to be dynamic.

The more congruent your intention, the more your energy will be focused on losing weight. Intention is defined as; *determination to act in some particular manner*. This determination to act purposefully can only come about if you truly want to lose weight; if you believe that you will attain your vision, and if you are prepared to accept that which you desire. You are most probably saying, "But of course I want to lose weight". But quite often we say we want something, but at a deeper level we resist this change. Be clear about your intention 'to have' that which you seek. Intention is linked to belief. We all have limiting beliefs, and it is these hidden beliefs that insidiously deny our ability to attain.

Beliefs like; "I'm not worthy of being loved", "I do not have it in me to achieve", "Life is unfair", or, "I have no control over my desires", are some examples of core beliefs that stand in the way of attaining weight loss.

Before you read on, spend some time reflecting on any limiting core-beliefs you may have. Write them down.

....
....
....
....

Now replace these limiting beliefs with positive beliefs that affirm your ability to attain. Write these down.

....
....
....
....
....

There may be times when you are visualizing, that you find that your energy is blocked. No matter how hard you try to visualize your 'slim body', you just can't seem to create a clear picture. This impediment can be due to a number of fundamental reasons. If it is because you are simply trying too hard, drop what you are attempting to do, relax and come back to visualizing when you feel more energized. Obsession is another form of 'over efforting'. As much as you have been encouraged to be inspired, to emotionally back up your intentions, and to involve yourself as much as possible in the process of creatively visualizing, there is one rider that needs to be added: there is no need to become obsessed about losing weight. As much as you may desire to lose weight - your desire to lose weight should not be so overwhelming that you become obsessive. Being too emotionally attached to any desire is an impediment to achieving your goal.

Recognize that any blockage at a deeper level is presenting you with an opportunity to address something about yourself that you have failed to pay attention to in the past. Blockages can be freed by observing and experiencing them. Blockages only have power while they remain hidden. They can only operate in darkness. Shining the light of awareness on them dissipates their power. Self-love and acceptance assists in releasing blocked energy.[10]

When you first begin practising creative visualization you may find that your old thought patterns are still determining your reality. There is often a time lag between the new thoughts you have put out and their manifestation. Thoughts exist in time. So, often those old thought patterns take some time to clear. You will find that as you become clearer on your in

---

[10] See Chapter 5 THE BEAUTY OF SELF

tentions your new thoughts will manifest quicker. In a way, this is life's means of allowing you to test the waters before new matters are realized. Do not allow this to deter you from practising creative visualization, for expansive thinking is an innately effective process that can effortlessly assist you in creating and realizing your dreams.

The ideal situation for visualizing is to be in a relaxed state. But you can also use to great effect, the 'mini-visualization'. This is when your time is limited. There are many opportunities during the day to use your time creatively. You can, for example prac-tice visualizing while you exercise. If you go to gym try visualizing each body part while cycling. See and feel the shape of your calves, thighs, abdomen, hips. Put your mind into your muscles and feel your shape beginning to change. Affirm the link between mind and body. See and feel your new slim figure. You can visualize while you are sitting on the bus, or in any situation where you have a few moments to spare. Use your spare time productively to enrich your life.

The more you practice visualization the greater your results will be. At first, you may consider setting aside specific times for visualizing. The best times are usually early morning on rising, midday, or just before going to bed. By setting regular times you strengthen the process of creating a new way of thinking and living. The more you practice and trust your visualizations the greater the results will be. You will be surprised at how easy it is to use creatively visualization for all areas of your life.

Creative visualization concerns consciously focusing on that which you wish to create or attain.

Often that which you wish to attain is frustrated by situations where something happens that causes you to respond in a reactive way. Someone says, or does something that you dislike. These particular situations arouse feelings and responses of an enervating nature. As you are aware, thoughts create feelings, and feelings determine responses. Our eating patterns are directly linked to what we feel. Besides genuine hunger signals, we generally overeat when we are unclear about issues (this may in some instances also manifest as a loathing for food - like anorexia or bulimia). It is interesting to note that emotions that create feelings of despondency, frustration, anger and the like, are always associated with a sense of helplessness. If you look beyond the emotion you will discover that you feel as though you do not have choice - that there is nothing that you can do to change the situation. In most instances you most probably feel that you are unable to confront the person or the issue; you do not believe you possibly have the resources to deal with the issue. Anger, jealousy, fear, anxiety, - all these emotions underline a sense of 'helplessness'.

It is therefore essential if you wish to lose weight, that you are able to direct your responses. This leads us to consider how you create your thought pictures and how it is possible to re-frame these pictures so that your thoughts arouse responses that support you in your quest to lose weight.

Re-Framing your Thought Pictures

Neurolinguistic Programming points out that each of us has our own 'strategy' for forming thought pictures. In other words we organize our images in a distinct way. The way in which you create *your* images determines your response to situations. As 'thoughts are things' they have the power to determine results. It is therefore vital that you are able to direct your thoughts. What do we mean when we say that each of us forms thought pictures in our own unique way?

You may for instance, when thinking about situations that you regard as pleasurable, tend to visualize the situation in images that are large and in colour.[11] Additionally your picture may also contain sound and motion. On the other hand, your response to unfavourable situations may elicit mental pictures that are comprised of small images in black and white, as opposed to the large and colourful images of your agreeable experiences. You may also see your images in the centre of your forehead, or to the left, or right of your brain. Someone else will compose their 'favourable' and 'unfavourable' images quite differently. What is important though, is that you should discover how **you** create your images - both 'favourable' and 'unfavourable'. There are no right or wrong ways to mentally visualize. Whatever works for you, is what is right.

The easiest way to discover how you access mental images is to do an exercise where you visualize a recent situation that excited or pleased you. Close your eyes and 'see' how you create your picture. Take note of what you see. Are the images that come up for you, large or small, in colour, or in black and white? Are they static, or do they have movement like a movie? Now take a situation that depresses you, and do the same exercise. You will notice that you have a completely different 'strategy' for your negative experiences.

Now, I would like you to take the situation that recently thrilled or excited you, and change your mental picture. If for example your initial images were

---

[11] For further reading see *Unlimited Power* by Anthony Robbins published by Simon and Schuster

large and bold, make them small. If they contained colour, make them black and white. If your picture contained sound, replace it with silence. Now, notice how your feelings have changed.

Do the same with your unfavourable experience. Think of a situation that recently made you depressed. Focus on those images that come up for you and alter them. If for example, your images were small and in black and white, expand them. Bring in colour and sound. You will notice that your feelings change as your picture changes. And, as your feelings change so do your responses.

Experiment with your images. Change the quality of your mental pictures and notice how your feelings change accordingly. With a bit of practice you will be able to effectively turn an unpleasant experience into an enabling experience.

The connection between what you think and what you experience determines what you will or will not achieve. The ability to re-frame will enable you to decisively broaden your ability to make choices that are energized and enabling.

As much as we are concerned with our conscious actions and their power to determine our future, there is another powerful connective aspect that warrants consideration, and that is, our ever present subconscious mind.

The Subconscious Mind

When it comes to the mind we are generally inclined to recognize the conscious mind. But there is another aspect to the holistic mind that is often neglected, namely the intelligent, perceptive, and ever-present subconscious mind.[12] It is often assumed that only the powers of reason and logic are capable of solving problems and providing creative insight. Yet, there is a point at which even the intelligence of the all-powerful conscious mind is limited by its functions.

It is normally thought that the subconscious mind is inaccessible due to the fact that it functions at a subliminal level and manifests in supposed arcane 'Freudian' ways. The Oxford Dictionary defines 'subconscious', as that part of the mind that is *"considered to be not fully conscious but able to influence actions"*.

The subconscious mind is capable of revealing much that is often not part of the process of conscious thought. The conscious mind functions on the basis of selection, generalization, and discrimination; where-as the subconscious mind absorbs and assimilates information inclusively without any preference. It literally soaks up all your impressions.

On the other hand the conscious mind only selects information on the basis of what it perceives to be important at the time. This selective aspect of the conscious mind is most apparent in the fact that shared experiences when compared are inevitably portrayed differently by each individual. Each witness presents their own version of what happened! This tendency to

---

[12] For the purpose of clarity, no distinction is made between the terms; subconscious or unconscious mind. 'Subconscious' is a term of popular psychology. Though frequently used as a synonym for 'unconscious' it is not equivalent to *unconscious* in Freudian theory, primarily because it blurs the distinction between unconscious and *preconscious*. Moreover, though apt to be associated with the psychology of Jung, it is not equivalent, either, to Jung's concept of the *collective unconscious*. - *The Fontana Dictionary of Modern Thought*.

'edit' what we experience, means that often we are incapable of seeing the full picture.

The subconscious mind does not have the capacity to rationalize nor does it selectively omit seemingly irrelevant aspects. It absorbs and assimilates the whole experience. The overriding character of the subconscious mind is its tendency to be totally explicit in its revelations. This is most evident in our dreams. Dreams reveal at both a literal, and symbolical level that which we have not consciously noticed, or that which we have chosen to ignore. Dreams present us with both the agreeable, and disagreeable aspects of our experience. They impart much that is valuable and often vital for personal growth.

Through dreams, subtle suggestion, creative images, and symbols, the subconscious mind is capable of revealing and communicating that which has been missed by the conscious activity of thought, providing necessary creative and insightful input.

The subconscious mind is defined both by its individual and collective nature. Carl Jung talked of the 'world soul' - the collective unconscious. The collective unconscious is everything each individual or race has ever experienced. The ability to draw on this infinite body of intelligence that transcends personal experience, gives the subconscious mind access to a pool of ideas and intelligence that is unlimited in its scope and potential. The attribution of the power of the collective subconscious to breakthroughs and discoveries in science, the arts, and many personal areas of experience are well documented. Some of the most seminal discoveries that have enabled mankind to move forward in its quest for attainment have been attributed to this innate form of intelligence. Thomas Edison (1847 - 1931), the archetypal American inventor who by the age of twenty one years had taken out over

1,000 patents is said to have slept in his laboratory in order to avail himself of any inspirational insights that came to him through his dreams and sub-conscious suggestions. His inventions ranged from automatic telegraph systems to electric lighting.[13] Another scientist, Nikola Tesla, recorded a vision he had of how electricity could be generated from waterfalls. Some twenty years later this vision of hydroelectricity was realized with a dynamo at Niagara Falls.[14]

At a personal level the subconscious mind is capable of assisting you in the many varied situations you face daily. This repository of wisdom and intelligence can be tapped by recognizing that the subconscious mind is a vital aspect of, and complement to, your conscious mind. Acknowledgement of this is the gateway to receiving assistance from your subconscious mind. Simply by putting out a request, going to your subconscious mind and asking for help, you open yourself up to receiving guidance. Normally the best times for invoking the assistance of your subconscious mind is during meditation, prayer, or before dropping off to sleep at night. Phrase your re-quest as simply as possible. You can ask for strength, succour, creative inspiration, or answers to your problems. If there is something you are struggling with at a personal level, request guidance on this issue. At some point during the ensuing days, you will in some subtle way be presented with your request. This can be in the form of dream revelation, creative images, symbols, or simply in the form of a deep abiding feeling.

Consideration of the subconscious mind and its relation to human potential constitutes an extensive and dynamic body of knowledge. Full consideration

---

[13] *The Oxford Reference Dictionary*
[14] *The Mind's Best Work* by D.N.Perkins Harvard University Press

would form the basis of another book. What is evident though at a fundamental level, is that the subconscious mind forms a powerful tool for self-attainment. The fact that the subconscious mind is non-judgemental (and is functional 24 hours a day) contains a double-edged implication: as much as it is predisposed to present you with unbiased information, it is incapable of discrimination. Whatever you tell it, it will accept. If you tell yourself that you are a failure, and that you can never succeed in losing weight, then your subconscious mind simply accepts this statement. It literally acts this out as failure! The conscious directives that are given to the subconscious mind are faithfully acted out.

It is this facet of the subconscious mind that holds such enormous potential for self-attainment - the power of suggestive self-affirmations. As you move through your day you are constantly talking to yourself, whether you are aware of this or not. You are constantly telling yourself what you think, and feel about your experiences and interactions. These self-statements are absorbed and retained by your subconscious mind for future use. They form powerful directives that are subliminally put into action.

If you tell yourself, "I am thin", then the message you are passing on to your body is "be thin". Your subconscious mind does not interpret this as; "He/she really does not know what he/she is talking about!". It responds literally to the directive it receives from the conscious mind. In turn, the electro-chemical message the body receives is; "Be thin!". Conversely, if what you say to yourself is, "I am fat", or, "I am useless", or any other self deprecating remark, then you can be assured that your subconscious mind will believe this, and you will manifest that which you have put out.

The statements you make magnetize and create what is going to happen to you.

Much of your communication to yourself concerns self-statements. These self-statements which form part of the stream of your inner monologue, determine how you will act out your future, - they determine the subconscious mental connection. The quality of your self-statements is that they either empower, or they limit you; they either affirm, or they deny your being.

The basis to all our self-statements are words. Words derive their power by association. In our minds we link words to images that we associate with past experiences, whether they be favourable or unfavourable. Words trigger off powerful associative images, especially if they are backed up by strong emotive feelings. Say to yourself; "I hate my fat body". Now express this self-statement with emotion, and it becomes a powerful directive that will not only elicit a limiting behavioral pattern, but it will also similarly program your subconscious mind. There is no way you can feel inclined to lose weight when you communicate this kind of self-statement. In fact, this type of limiting self-statement will direct you straight back to the actions that created the situation in the first place. Let us examine another self-statement that you might make while running or exercising: "I am filled with energy". On one level this affirmative self-statement communicates empowering feelings to your body, which in turn gives you the wherewithal to stretch yourself that bit more. At another level, the subconscious mind receives input that unequivocally validates your ability to achieve. As it does not have the capacity to discern whether you mean what you say or not, it acts this out as an enabling action. Your subconscious mind is literally programmed by your inner communication. How you communicate with yourself determines your outcome.

It is therefore of consequence that you become aware of the statements you make to yourself. As you move through your day pay attention to the way in which you talk to yourself, and your choice of words. Remember everything you tell yourself is acted on, for your subconscious mind is unable to discriminate.

Self-affirmations send positive messages to your mind. When you feel down on yourself because you are not losing weight fast enough, or you find it difficult to view yourself differently, or change your eating patterns, endorse your potentiality through affirmative self-statements. Support your intention to lose weight by becoming aware of the limiting self-statements you make. Replace them with positive and enabling self-statements.

Exercise

Take note of some of the self-limiting statements you repeatedly make to yourself:

....

....

....

....

As you become aware of your limiting self-statements, substitute them for empowering self-statements. It is much easier and takes far less energy to be positive, than negative. Tom Kubistant, Ed.D. in his book Mind

Pump, states "…. *The physiological and psychological sciences have recently confirmed that the body and mind are designed to be positive."*

Ponder for a few moments the outcome of replacing your self-limiting statements with powerful self-empowering statements. Consider the situation where virtually every statement and thought you think affirms every aspect of your being. It doesn't take much imagination to realize the potentiality of this. If every thought, every statement was positive, you would, in a short matter of time begin to attain your visions and intentions. You would manifest what you think and believe. This possibility is certainly not wishful thinking. It is a certainty! It all depends on your input. In the computer world there is a saying; "Garbage in, Garbage out". The same applies to your mind. Therefore, quality input = quality output. You deserve the best. Send your subconscious mind statements of excellence. One of the simplest and most potent ways of doing this, is through *self-affirmations.*

Self-Affirmations

Affirmations are positive assertions we make to ourselves. They are powerful statements about our potential and capabilities. Affirmations confirm our belief in ourselves. You can say affirmations out aloud, or quietly to yourself. Written down they reinforce your intention to achieve. What is important is that you focus on what you want, not on what you do not want. If you focus on what you don't want, that is what you will get! By making the self-statement, "I don't want to be fat", you are sending your subconscious mind a contradictory message. The only way you can experience this self-statement is by being fat. It is like saying; "I do not want to fail". The only way your mind can experience this, is by failing!

The self-statements; "I am thin", or, "I am losing weight", state clearly that you are empowered. "I don't want to be overweight", says; "I really do not know what I want, and I really do not believe that I have the power to lose weight".

The stronger your belief, the greater the power of the affirmation. The feeling that backs your self-statement gives propulsion to the thought. Get a sense of your power to create. Repetition reinforces this new belief in yourself and backs up your memory.[15] The more frequently you repeat your empowering affirmations, the more they become part of your subconscious mind. The affirmations you choose should always feel comfortable. Find affirmations that feel natural and right for you. Any resistance you feel will dissipate the clarity and punch of your statement. There may be times that you experience resistance to a new affirmation. This may merely be the ego under threat. If this feeling persists, re-frame your affirmation or replace it with another self-empowering statement.

The other important point to remember, is to always phrase your statements in the present tense. Constructing your statements in the future carries suggestions of indecisiveness and wishful thinking. Rather than saying to yourself, "I will lose weight"; say "I am losing weight", or "My body is firm and lean".

---

[15] *The subconscious mind functions as a memory bank for storing our experiences. Like all data banks, these experiences and perceptions are filed away according to their pattern. In the process, they are converted over time into concepts - that either empower or limit us. Memory thus acts as a filter, colouring and determining our responses.* From Voluntary Controls by Jack Schwarz published by Penguin Arkana

Statements that are short and to the point are more effective than long drawn out constructions which tend to lose their clarity and force.

Experiment with new affirmations. What works for you at this point in time may not meet your changing future needs. Remember you are continually developing; nothing remains the same. Attune your affirmations to your evolving needs.

There are basically two types of affirmations: general and specific.

General Affirmations

General affirmations relate to the broad areas of your life. Here are a few:
"I love myself more each day".
"I am in control of my life".
"The more I understand the more I attain".
"I am the centre of my energy".
"Everything I need is within".
"I am a radiant and loving person".
"I am beautiful and vital".
"I'm excited by my potential to create".
"I love myself as I am".
"I am a powerful and loving being".
"I express myself freely and fully".

Now fill in some of your own general affirmations that will affirm your right to lose weight and attain your vision:

....
....

Specific Affirmations

Specific affirmations are directed towards certain definite areas of your life. Eating, exercising, working, or personal relationships are areas where you would use specific affirmations. You can say one of the following affirmations, or if none of these work for you, make up one that feels right for you:

"I am slim and firm".
"I have a great figure".
"I have great calves".
"My metabolism works for me".
"My body is beautiful ".
"I eat only what my body needs".

Fill in those specific affirmations that will empower you to lose weight:

....

....

....

....

Repeat these affirmations to yourself. Feel the vigour and energy of these self-statements. Use both types of affirmations to assist you in losing weight and changing your eating patterns. Expand these affirmations into all areas of your life.

You may elicit greater inspiration and assurance by also including referrals to spiritual sources when you create you affirmations. If you believe that the universal creative energy manifests as God, Christ, Buddha, Allah, All-That-Is, the Light, or any other spiritual source, use this to enhance your affirmation.

You may use:
"Divine love helps me create what I need".
"God's love guides my thoughts".
"God assists me in everything I do".
"I draw on the universal energy".

Repeat your affirmations as often as you can. Use them to endorse your power to lose weight.

What are the principal points you have learnt about affirmations?

....

....

....

....

What uplifting affirmation are you going to start using **now** to lose weight?

....

....

....

The Emotional Body

You may not have ever heard Richard Burton, or Martin Luther King move their audience, but if you have heard a powerful speaker arouse his audience then you have experienced the power of emotional energy. This power can move people to tears, or arouse them to pick up arms and go to war. The root of emotion is derived from the Latin word *movere*, which means 'to move'. Statements like, "I hate my body", or "I love food", are all expressions of *"e-motion - energy in motion"*.[16] They carry with them the power to affect your response to situations; ultimately, they determine the results you create.

Emotions can cut both ways; they can cause devastation or they can be totally uplifting. If not channelled they can cause havoc in your life and relationships. Like a torrent of water, the stream of emotion needs to be directed to be of benefit.

Just as the mind uses the brain to realize its intentions, so your emotional body uses the heart for the expression of higher emotions. Love, compassion, and devotion are all expressions of the heart. It is these emotions that give one a sense of inner harmony and illumination. Emotions like anger, hatred, jealousy and resentment emanate from the solar plexus and are of a different nature to those of the heart.

It is easy to distinguish between these different types of emotions: the next time you are stressed-out, locate where these feelings are coming from. The knot in your solar plexus is a telling sign of a base emotion. On the other hand, heart emotions which are located higher up in the body, have the ennobling qualities of

---

[16] *The Power of the Heart* by Sara Paddison published by Planetary Publications.

upliftment. Heart emotions fill you with a pervasive feeling of harmonious accord. The heart has the innate intelligence of bringing balance and understanding into your life and is the key to attaining harmony between the mind and those runaway emotions that cause conflict and opposition. Connect-ing with the heart gives you a focus that can dissolve those restive feelings of anger, fear, and depression that so often stand in the way of attaining weight loss, happiness, or any other personal goal.

Fat Equals Thin!

If you are overweight, this is proof that your ability to emotionally respond is highly developed. The fact that you may not have used some of these responses to validate your right to be THIN, in no way denies your capacity to direct your emotions. Understanding 'how' you elicit your emotions, is the key to losing weight and finding fulfilment.

Transmuting Emotion

As you go about your day, situations arise where certain thoughts cause you to react in an emotionally obstructive manner. The typical scenario usually reads something like this: during the course of the day someone says, or does something that affects you. This causes you to become upset, or angry. As the day progresses you mentally keep coming back to the situation. The more you mull over the issue in your mind, the more your base emotions well up. Discord grows with each successive attempt to mentally deal with the issue. Finally, the only way you can find release is through some form of excessive behaviour.

There are of course a number of other alternatives to resolving this type of mental/emotional loop. One of the choices you can make in attempting to resolve the situation is to confront the source of the problem - in this case, the person with which you had the disagreement. Failing this, your next choice is more often than not to seek solace through self-gratification. Food or drink usually fulfils this demand. But as we all know so well, any situation that requires a trade-off, comes at a price. Excessive behaviour in the form of overeating or any other indulgence, inevitably leads to some consequence - generally becoming overweight, or ill health. Yet, as much as we are inclined at times to respond negatively to certain situations there is another way of dealing with these emotional issues.

There is within all of us the means to effortlessly right any imbalance that we may manifest. Our base emotions that operate through the solar plexus are connected to the heart. This connection enables the heart to transmute these emotions into harmonious higher emotions. Redirecting your energy through your heart enables you to access the power and intelligence of the heart - herein lies the freedom of choice.

At this point it is necessary appreciate that, 'base' emotions are not necessarily negative. There are certain situations where base emotions are appropriate. If your life were threatened, fear or anger may very well serve you in this situation. At other times, these very same emotions add to the turmoil and stress in your life. The important aspect to appreciate is that self-empowerment denotes the ability to make choices: to determine what best suits your varying needs and to be able to direct your life rather than be blown about like a kite in the sky on a gusty day.

What happens when you feel negative towards yourself? How do you re-direct these disempowering feelings? How do you work through the depression, the anger, the fear, or whatever other limiting feelings you experience? How do you release those emotional blocks that stand in the way of self-fulfilment?

Lets take the self-statement, "No matter how hard I try, I never seem to lose weight". The emotion that backs this can be so insidious as to limit your ability to lose weight. It can stand between you and what you truly desire. When you express a base emotion (solar plexus) you respond to this feeling by firstly believing it to be an entity, a 'thing' that stands apart from you. You fail to recognize that it is merely a state of mind that you have chosen to express. The resentment you feel also convinces you that this 'thing' must be real and that it must have substance. The effect of all this is that your emotional state now generates thoughts that send your subconscious mind the message that you do not have the ability to succeed. And, without question, after all the effort you have put into failing, there is no way you are going to succeed in losing weight. How then do you work through these situations that so inhibit your ability to achieve?

Firstly, it is necessary to acknowledge that feelings are of such a nature that they are usually too strong to suppress. Once you are in an 'emotional state', it does not help to attempt to replace debilitating emotions with so called 'positive' emotions. As we all know, once you are caught up in an emotionally destructive state, it is not possible to suddenly start feeling proactive. Instead, it is far more prudent to become a disinterested **observer**. Simply allow these feelings to be. Experience the sensations they produce. Then, shift your attention to your heart. You will find that in this process that something subtly begins to shift. You will pass through the tumultuous emotional level of the experience and into the real energy that exists behind it. It is in this discovery that you begin to transmute those base emotions. It is in this process that your heart begins to transmute feelings of inadequacy, resentment, anger, depression etc., into tender feelings of love, compassion and understanding. It is the admixture of love that releases the healing power of the heart.

If you feel fearful about looking at your emotions, recognize that you may feel that your base emotions are in some way unacceptable. As already mentioned, all forms of emotion serve a purpose. In the appropriate situation, the appropriate response is fitting. By acknowledging that every base emotion serves a need, that there is a context within which this response is appropriate, you allow your heart to present you with other options. This approach enables you to have choice. Denial, suppression, and judgement only strengthens resistance to change. When you come from your heart, when you feel love and compassion for yourself, you have no need to compare or judge your thoughts or emotions. By its very nature, love seeks accord and union. By going to the heart you gain a perspective that enables you to find fulfilment and harmony. The intelligence of the heart takes you away from the anger and judgement of the mind. It is no wonder that all the great spiritual and religious teachers have emphasised the power of the heart. Their admonishment to go to the heart and be filled with love in times of anger and hatred, is based on a profound wisdom of the healing power of the heart.

The heart is the key to achieving balance in your life. What is often missed, is that all forms of power need to be qualified, to be balanced in a way that enables us to achieve a measure of excellence.

Preoccupation with the development of the intellect, without the corresponding inclusion of compassion and love, is a prescription for personal disorder and dysfunction.

Balance is necessary for the functioning of wellbeing. The wisdom of the heart can add a dimension that intuitively offers you a deep intelligence, for the head and the heart are intended to act together - in harmonious unison. In times of personal distress you can access your heart power by linking directly with your heart. Placing your focus on the heart redirects your energy. You can always rely on your heart to give you the truth. For the heart has no inclination to distort or deceive. When love is turned into obsession or attachment, it is not the heart that deforms the feeling of love, but rather the machinations of the mind that twists this virtue. The distinction of the heart is that it neither judges, compares, nor blames - these are the very acts of mind, not heart.

As you go about your day practice going to the heart, familiarize yourself with the feelings of this judicious centre. You will soon discover the sense of tranquillity, peace and ease that these feelings produce. Place your energy and attention on the heart area. Visualize the heart as your centre of expansion and love. In her book "Working with the Chakras" Ruth White describes spring green, rose and rose amethyst as the colours of the heart. She tells us that visualizing the colour spring green as you focus on the heart area, assists in opening up the heart and healing old hurts. Concentrating on the colour rose promotes a sense of solace and serenity. If you have been afflicted by illness or stress, focusing on the colour of rose amethyst will strengthen the heart.

Affirmations are connective links that also assist in harmonizing your emotions. A very effective affirmation that you can say to yourself is: *"In the golden centre of the rose of the heart, may tender compassion be linked to unconditional love."* [17] As you work with the harmonizing energies of the heart you will find that you will strengthen your heart connection. The more you are able to connect, the more you will be able to move from lesser emotional issues to far deeper emotional issues. The ability to re-direct emotion, forms one aspect of emotion. The other, concerns the ability of being able to elicit enabling emotions.

How do you elicit an enabling state of emotion, and is it possible to evoke emotions that lead to fulfilment and joy? Just as you create anger, fear, or any other base emotion through certain mental attitudes and physiological responses, so you create enabling emotions.

The next time you experience emotions (base emotions) that propel you to overeat, take note of what you say to yourself. Notice the tone of voice you use, and your choice of words. Become aware of the visual images you construct in your mind. Similarly, take note of your physical demeanour: Do you adopt a posture that indicates that you are energized, or do you adopt a posture of someone that is in a slump? What are your breathing patterns? Every detail of what you do will give you vital clues as to how you effectively create a state of depression, anger, or any other emotion. Now, if you wish to effectively create emotions that back up your intention to lose weight, all you need to do is to change the modalities of your strategy. In place of telling yourself that you are a failure, that you are unable to lose weight rather affirm that you have the capability and potential to lose all the weight you need. Instead of picking up emotions that do not

---

[17] *Working with your Chakras* by Ruth White, published by Piatkus.

benefit you, come from the heart. Move the energy from your solar plexus up into your heart. Suffuse your being with self-love. Check out your physical demeanour; if need be flaunt the posture of assurance, push your shoulders back, lift your head up and walk with the gait of someone who feels great about themself. Whatever strategy you successfully employed to create an emotional state that brings you down - the same strategy will work for lifting you up. Change the modalities of your strategy and you will be surprised at the results.

It is also interesting to note that *"Biochemists have discovered that as a result of experiencing positive emotions powerful pituitary proteins and peptides are produced which can induce a state of pleasure in the body".*[18] Revealing research by Dr Candace Pert, chief of brain biochemistry at the National Institute of Noetic Sciences makes some of the following find-ings in her article titled "Neuropeptides: The Emotions and Bodymind"[19]

"Recent research suggests that neuropeptides (chemical substances made and released by the brain cells and certain other cells) may provide the key to an understanding of the body's chemistry of emotion. They appear to serve as a newly discovered form of communication within the body.....I believe that neuropeptides and their receptors are a key to understanding how mind and body are interconnected and how emotions can manifest throughout the body. Dr. Pert argues that the three classic areas of neuroscience, endocrinology, and immunology, with their various organs - the brain

---

[18] *Ultrahealth* by Lesley Kenton published by Protea Paperbacks.
[19] Article adapted by Harris Dienstfrey from a talk delivered at the Symposium on Consciousness and Survival sponsored by the Institute of Noetic Sciences, October 25/26, 1985.

(which is the key organ that the neuroscientists study), the glands, and the immune system (consisting of the spleen, the bone marrow, the lymph nodes, and of course the cells circulating through the body) - that these three areas are actually joined to each other in a bi-directional network of communication and that the information 'carriers' are the neuropeptides. Dr. Candace Pert's research advances that emotions have the ability to affect one's health. Neuropeptides (chemical substances that are produced by the brain in repsonse to emotional activity) somehow communicate with the body's immune system. Some of these findings are paraphrased below.

Monocytes, which are pivotal in the immune system, are cells with vital health-sustaining functions. Monocytes are responsible not just for recognising and digesting foreign bodies, but also for wound-healing and tissue-repair mechanisms. A monocyte travels along in the blood and at some point comes within "scenting" distance of a neuropeptide, and because the monocyte has receptors for the neuropeptide on it's cell surface, it begins literally to chemotax, or crawl toward that chemical. Neuropeptides and other emotion-affecting bio-chemicals appear to control the routing and migration of monocytes. They communicate and interact in the whole system to fight disease and to distinguish between self and non-self, deciding, say, which part of the body is a tumour cell to be killed by natural killer cells, and which parts need to be restored. It turns out that the cells of the immune system not only have receptors for these various neuropeptides; they also make the neuropeptides themselves.

Ernest Rossi in The Psychobiology of Mind-Body Healing goes on to say: *"This messenger molecule (neuropeptide) and cell-receptor communication system is the psychobiological basis of mind-body healing, therapeutic hypnosis, and holistic medicine in general."*

Although scientific research has only just begun to make inroads into the chemistry of emotion, the indications are that emotions can no longer be regarded in an elementary way. Neuropeptide receptor sites appear to be located throughout the body and are vitally connected to the body as whole. This 'interconnectedness' impinges not only on our emotional states, but also on our very well-being and health. From these astonishing findings it can be assumed that enabling emotions somehow have an inordinate capacity to heal. One need only look at someone who is in love to see the benefit of the emotions of the heart. They radiate beauty and well-being. If you have ever attempted to lose weight when you were in love, then you will know how easy it is to lose all that unwanted weight. On the other hand, try and lose weight when your are depressed! Look at someone who is embittered; not only are they affected by these feelings, but even their faces are etched with lines of anger and bitterness.

Emotion is a vital link between mind and body. Emotions give a range of expression and colour to the physical body that can be directed through self-awareness. When channelled effectively emotion acts as an uplifting force to mind, body, and spirit.

The Emotional Loop!

Emotions are generally connected to thoughts. Every thought that attempts to evaluate, classify, or measure a situation involves judgement. Judgement implies 'good' or 'bad', 'right' or 'wrong', 'like' or 'dislike'. Any judgement must evoke some form of emotional response. So, the pattern to identify is; thoughts evoke feelings, feelings influence your responses, and responses determine results!

The Physical Body

As the seed is within the banyan tree,
and within the seed are the flowers,
the fruits, and the shade;
so the germ is within the body,
and within that germ is the body again.
.....The lifespark is hidden in your body - the germ that can become a flowering, the seed that can become God - the potentiality is hidden in the body. Don't fight with it, because the potentiality is very fragile: if you fight the body you will destroy that potentiality. The body has to be looked after.

Kabir (15th.Century Poet/Mystic)

Certainly one of the most awe-inspiring of all the universe's wonders must be the human body. Consider how your body is capable of creating life, or the body's miraculous capacity to heal itself. If you but only fleetingly reflect on any of the body's functions, then you must acknowledge that of all Earth's marvels, your body is one of the most phenomenal.

As the poet mystic Kabir states in the above passage, *"The lifespark is hidden in your body ..... the seed that can become God."* Through your body and your senses you are able to connect the outer with inner. Your ability to conceptually, perceptually, and emotional experience is possible only through the your bodily senses.

The body is your feedback mechanism. Whatever you think, feel, or express, is revealed through your body. It is your mirror. The body responds directly to the stimuli it receives. Think FAT, and you will become fat. Emotionally respond with continual self-depleting feelings and you will affect your body's immune system. Eat badly and your body will render this as overweight, ill health, and a lack of energy. But nurture your body, give it mental, physical, emotional, and spiritual nourishment and it will respond munificently - yielding health, energy and self-fulfilment.

I am always amazed at how much abuse our bodies are capable of handling. Despite all this our bodies continue to support us, albeit at a less than optimal level. The body's inherent inclination is to assure that you experience fulfilment. It is predisposed to function optimally, to replace and repair tissue cells, to heal and uplift. At a cellular level it is infused not only with the need to survive, but to ensure expansive ennoblement. This ennoblement embraces mental, physical, emotional, and spiritual fulfilment.

The physical body is vitally dependant on nutritional nourishment for its survival. At the most basic level, deprivation of food and water inevitably leads to death. At the most elevated level, nutritional fulfilment assures glowing health, a well proportioned firm figure, and general well-being. The aphorism, *you are what you eat,* is certainly reflected in one's body. The inevitable question must therefore be asked: What constitutes optimum nutrition? What do you need to eat to ensure that you not only lose weight, but that you enjoy a state of physical well-being? The question of nutrition begets the need to first examine the fundamental issue of 'you' - the individual.

The thrust of losing weight, health, beauty, or any other form of fulfilment is based on the harmonious alignment of your four bodies and the recognition that each individual is inherently unique. The fact that we all have the same organs and essential biochemical functions, does not preclude the fact that our personal (mental, physical, emotional and spiritual) needs differ. In order to effect effortless and lasting weight loss it is necessary to embrace the understanding that your body's needs are unique and distinctive. As your body is affected by what you eat, so too it is affected by your thoughts, emotions, and spiritual responses. The recognition of your body's diverse and varying needs therefore necessitates an intuitive awareness that transcends the limitations of a rigid dietary approach.

Rather than prescribing what you should eat or how you should live, it is far more important that you are empowered to respond intuitively and effectively to your varying needs and conditions. Time alone verifies the illusion of constancy. Neither you nor the universe remains fixed: each moment the shift of time underscores the need for attentive awareness to perpetual change. And, within this change lies the marvel and the mystery of the moment - and the ever new.

This recognition inevitable leads us to face the issue of what constitutes an intuitional approach to nutrition. The subject of this forms the basis to Chapter Seven - Eating for Pleasure. At this point though, it is only necessary that you begin to recognize that your nutritional needs are not unvarying, - that you are essentially dynamic in all aspects of your being.

Body Awareness Exercise

Before you proceed with this section spend a few minutes focusing on the most wondrous universal creation - your body. Try and get a sense of the divine gift that you are endowed with. Take a few deep breaths and become aware of your body, feel the beat of your heart, the rhythm of your breathing. Extend this awareness to your senses of sight, sound, taste, smell, and touch. This is best done by beginning with your visual sense. Block your ears and focus only on seeing. Now close your eyes and become aware of sound. Keeping your eyes closed and your ears blocked, focus on your sense of smell. It is not that easy to isolate the senses of taste and touch, but with a little bit of imagination it is possible to appreciate just how important these senses are to your fulfilment.

As you go about your day try and extend this awareness to all of your activities. When you sit down to eat, see if you can retain this awareness. As you become more aware of your body you will begin to allow your body to tell you through its innate intelligence what your nutritional and other needs are.

The messages your body sends out need to be responded to in order to maintain an optimal state of function and vitality.[20] If your body is healthy, not only will you benefit mentally, but your skin will glow, your eyes sparkle, and your hair shine. You will radiate a sense of general well-being. Beauty therapy today acknowledges that external beauty is most directly achieved through good health - **health equals Beauty**.

The Power of Physiology

There is another exciting facet to the human body that is often not fully recognized and that is the power of physiology. Physical responses directly affect one's state of mind. As much as thoughts have the capacity to impact on your mannerisms, posture, breathing and general physical behaviour, so too physiology has the ability to impact neurologically on your mental states.

---

[20] These proprioceptive(internal) stimuli arise naturally from within the body itself and differ from those stimuli received from the senses.

Recent research has confirmed that physical actions produce electro-chemical responses in the brain. This suggestion opens up a vast potential that can be used to direct your physical resources to creating empowering states of mind.

How you 'act' in effect determines the messages you send to your brain. The power of physiology can be witnessed by simply looking around you. Have you ever seen a successful athlete or a dynamic achiever with the body language of an also-ran? Think back to times when you were successful, was your physiology vital or lethargic? Were your shoulders stooped and your eyes downcast? I'm willing to bet that your physiology was anything but one of self-deprecation. On the other hand, look at those who are always inclined to bemoaning their lot in life. The physiology of these people is as depressed as their state of mind. Anthony Robbins in his book titled *Unlimited Power*, clearly confirms the power of physiology in the chapter: *Physiology: The Avenue of Excellence* "....*The way you use your physiology - the way you breathe and hold your body, your posture, facial expressions, the nature and quality of your movements - actually determines what state you are in. The state you are in will then determine the range and quality of the behaviors you are able to produce.*"

There is a synergistic link between your physiology and your mental state. This link runs both ways, if the mind is depressed then the body is depressed; if the body is depressed the mind is depressed. Conversely, if the body is energized - the mind is energized. By becoming aware of how your body 'represents', you have the means to instantly change your mental state. If you do not believe this, start yawning and see what happens! All of a sudden you will start feeling tired and listless. Now strut your stuff: act like you are filled with a sense of your worth, push your shoulders back, effect the tilt of head that says; "Yes I have the what it takes to be able to direct my life". As you will discover, this action sets up an enabling chain. If you take on the body posture of assuredness you create a feeling of conviction. This feeling in turn creates an enabling state of mind which consequently allows you to effect a positive action. Turn this around and you have its opposite, a limiting sequence.

> ## *The Physiology Loop*
> *The way in which you physically 'represent', determines what you feel. In turn these feelings colour how you respond. And, how you respond determines the result you produce. So, as much as a 'THOUGHT LOOP' determines what you are capable of achieving, so a 'PHYSIOLOGICAL LOOP' determines the results you produce!*

When you feel capable of achieving, you are willing to put a foot forward. You are willing to explore new areas and change old habitual attitudes and responses. You can only begin changing your eating habits and beliefs when you are in an empowered state. If you feel unresourceful, you will be unresourceful - you will perpetuate the same old behavioral patterns.

Physiology is a pathway to effortless transformation. Change your physiology and you change your state of mind. It's a simple as that! The way in which you physiologically present has a corresponding capacity to affect your state of mind. When you next feel depressed or upset, take note of how you physically represent this emotional state. Remember to change your physiology. Visualize yourself as a dynamic and joyous person. Stand erect and push your shoulders out. Look up and take in deep strong breaths. Get a sense of your beauty and strength. You will find that immediately you change your physiology you will change the way you feel about yourself. And, when you feel great you act great.

Physiology is not only a link between your body and your mind, it is also a link between your emotions and behavioral patterns. Emotional states like depression, frustration and anger, are often coupled to the behavioral response of overeating. The next time you go on a 'Food Binge' take note of your physiology. Become aware of your posture, your breathing patterns - see if your body language is that of someone who is empowered, someone who feels good about themselves. You will be amazed at how 'literally' the body represents your inner mental and emotional states. By changing your physiology, you can simply and effectively change your responses. Physiology has the power to assist you in losing weight.

Fat Equals Thin!

If you successfully created yourself overweight - then as I am sure you are already beginning to realize; you must have used the power of physiology. So, turn this around, - back up your intentions to lose weight with the physiology of someone who is empowered- someone who has choice.

There is nothing complicated about connecting with the power of physiology. All that is required, is that you become aware of how this body/mind link either benefits or affects your ability to be effective. Awareness is the key to affirmatively orchestrating your physiology in support of your quest for self-attainment.

Finally, there is one more vital aspect that needs to be integrated in order to realize your full empowerment and potential, and that is the connective force between mind, body, and emotions - the essence to your being - your Spiritual Body.

The Spiritual Body

If you have ever sat quietly watching the waves endlessly roll onto the beach, or strolled through some wooded glade in an attempt to find a solution to some pressing problem; or if you have ever meditated or made an invocation to obtain clarity and understanding - then you have endeavored to attain the wisdom of your spiritual body, your Higher Self. Whether you attribute the source of this wisdom to God, All-That-Is, the Light, Christ-Consciousness, Buddha, or Allah - what you are alluding to is a source of power and intelligence that extends beyond what you are normally capable of accessing.

Your Higher Self is all-knowing, it is your wise inner teacher. Its wisdom and intelligence is not limited by conscious knowledge, time or subconscious memory. The dimensions of your Higher Self enable you to possess a far more expansive and profound view of matters than you would normally have. Your spiritual body is able to *"bring you a message of the nature of the whole; it partakes of the omniscience of universal mind"*[21]

---

[21] *Voluntary Controls - Exercises for Creative Meditation* by Jack Schwartz published by Penguin Arkana.

The wisdom of your Higher Self aligns and exalts all your bodies to form a more harmonious whole - it merges with mind, emotions, and physical body. As you learn to align with your Higher Self, you will enjoy benefits in all areas of your life: your mind will become more lucid, your emotions more harmonized and your body more vital. This connection will bring health, harmony, and an abiding love for both yourself and those around you. As you begin to trust in the wisdom of your Higher Self, you will become sensitive to the subtle energies of this intelligence. This awareness will expand your ability to bring about changes in all areas of your life.

Your Higher Self expresses its wisdom and intelligence in diverse ways: through intuition, feelings, inspiration, and visions. These insights, revelations, and inspired states of experience connect you with your source of deepest intelligence and wisdom. This profound knowing, this divine connection is evident in much of what you experience in your daily life. If you momentarily reflect you will recall having experienced at one time or another, the prompting of your Higher Self. It may have been a nagging unease about going ahead with something, which with hindsight proved to be correct. Or it may have been a situation where you felt impelled to do something that didn't seem to logically make sense at the time. Going with this feeling in the end proved to be the right choice. This assistance may also come in the form of coincidence; a chance meeting with some person, the acquisition of a book, or some accidental situation that reveals something that you need to know.

Your Higher Self enables you to experience yourself as the creator of your universe. Those moments of inspired clarity, vision and expanded wisdom that you experience from time to time, are all manifestations of your Higher Self.

Your Higher Self is connected to your personality self. In order to physically make changes to your body (lose weight) and improve your life, it is necessary that you develop this two way channel between your personality and your Higher Self. You can channel the wisdom of your Higher Self through requesting guidance on any matter. Answers needed to solve personal, health, or creative problems can all be realized through opening up to your Higher Self. There are numerous examples of seminal discoveries and creative breakthroughs being attributed to the Higher Self. Much has been written about Mozart's ability to artistically 'channel' his music. One such example is the overture to Don Giovanni; generally regarded as one of his best overtures. The overture was composed late the night before he was due to present his composition for performance. The story is told of Mozart having drunk prodigiously beforehand and having to be kept awake by his wife's conversation, all the while penning his masterpiece. In the early hours of the morning he finally fell asleep, his composition incomplete. At five o'clock in the morning he awoke, two hours before the music copyists were due to arrive. In the remaining time he was able to complete the overture just in time for the music sheets to be rushed to the awaiting orchestra. Henri Poincare, the French mathematician and philosopher of science who pioneered algebraic topology and contributed to the transformation of celestial mechanics is said to have regarded this form of intelligence as invaluable. William Blake, Elias Howe the inventor of the lockstich sewing machine, Albert Einstein, Charles Darwin and Marie Curie whose discoveries underpinned nuclear physics, are but a few of the luminaries that used insight, revelation, intuition and guidance as a means to further their work.

Requesting guidance involves stilling your mind, going within and creating that quiet space that enables insight to be channelled through your Higher Self. In this state you can request inspiration, solutions to problems, or advice. The wise guidance you receive often comes in the form of intuition, acute feelings, impressions, words, or mental images. One of the most effective ways of channelling your Higher Self is through meditation or invocation. You can also obtain guidance through incubating your request before going to sleep.[22] The following meditation is offered as one of the many ways in which you can access your higher power.

The Higher Self Meditation

Step 1

The first step in any form of meditation is being able to relax. As detailed in Chapter 3: Self-empowerment: The Mental Body; the deeper the relaxation, the greater the benefit. Relaxing enables you to slow down your brain-wave patterns, making you responsive to heightened awareness. To save you having to refer back to this section, the sequence on how to relax is repeated for your convenience.

Find a quiet spot either in your house or in your garden. We all have our 'power spots' where we feel

---

[22] Incubation simply means to request advice from your Higher Self to a specific issue or problem just before going to sleep. It is essential that you not only clarify your request, but that you also ensure that you are relaxed and mentally focused. Writing down your request on a piece of paper helps to elucidate and affirm your injunction.

particularly comfortable and energized. You should be able to relax and focus your mind without being disturbed either by your family or the telephone. Those of you that have meditated before will have already established your own approach to relaxing.

Sit in a comfortable position. Make sure that your spine is completely erect. Close your eyes and become aware of yourself...... Listen to the sounds, both those outside and inside of you .... Allow these sounds to pass through you.... Now become aware of your sense of smell..... Taste how your mouth feels...... Feel yourself becoming more centred.....Take a few deep breaths and as you exhale, imagine all your tension and worries leaving you .....Watch your breathing, feel its natural rhythm.

Now starting with the top of your head, work downward. Feel your face muscles beginning to relax.... Move down your neck and shoulders, feeling the tension draining away ......If you are distracted by thoughts or sounds, merely acknowledge their presence and continue. Move your attention through each part of your body.....down your thighs, knees, calves, ankles, feet and toes ...... Enjoy this feeling of relaxation.

Step 2

Visualize a white light moving up through your body. Feel this energy as it travels along your legs and up your spine to your head. Allow the white light to settle at a point on your forehead somewhere between your eyes - this is the region that is often referred to as your 'third eye'.

Step 3

Imagine a setting - this can be a timeless lunar landscape, a lush green mountain valley, an endless beach with the sun sinking below an orange horizon - create whatever setting works for you. Now picture your Higher Self coming towards you. You might visualize this as vibrant light, or as an image of yourself. This image may be a heightened and idealized representation of your full potentiality. Picture this image as clearly as possible. It is important that whatever you visualize feels comfortable. Experience the love and joy that your Higher Self radiates as it approaches. When your Higher Self finally reaches you, allow it to merge into your being. Feel the ex-pansive energy and wisdom that emanates from this connection.

Step 4

Think of your Higher Self as a wise oracle that knows all the answers to your questions. As your Higher Self you are going answer what you need to know. Your answer may come to you directly, or it may come you to later on in the form of an idea, suggestion, or dream.

Step 5

Acknowledge your Higher Self by thanking it. At any time in the future you can call on your Higher Self to provide you with further guidance and answers to your problems.

The wisdom and intelligence of your Higher Self not only functions in providing guidance, but serves to enable you to experience yourself as the co-creator of your universe. The source of your Higher Self is evident in whatever you can see, touch, feel, taste or hear - in fact whatever you are capable of perceptually, cognitively or emotionally experiencing is the result of the expression of ALL-THAT-IS.

"One might say that the finer substances and energies in the spiritual body induce harmonic resonance in the lower three bodies. This process continues all the way down into the frequency level of the physical body. Each body expresses this impulse in terms of its conscious reality at its own level".[23]

As such, the creative intelligence of All-That-Is is available to you through your Higher Self to be dynamically experienced through the expansiveness of your thoughts and feelings. When you are being expansive your Higher Self uplifts all aspects of your mental, emotional and physical expression.

Energy is the essence to all manifestation, whether it be divine or temporal. Energy is mutable and can be directed by what you think. When you attentively and expansively focus on your thoughts you are working with creative energy. This outflow comes from your Higher Self. The more expansive your thoughts, the more expansive the results. You can lose weight, enjoy radiant health or meet any other need by invoking your Higher Self.

As you connect with your Higher Self you will be able to access the answers and wisdom you need to deal with losing weight. You will also experience yourself in an expanded, vital and creative way. It is important that you understand that accessing your Higher Self is not something that needs to be developed. Your Higher Self is already fully developed - it is only the layers of conditioning, habitual response and

---

[23] *Hands of Light: A Guide to Healing through the Human Energy Field* by Barbara Ann Brennan published by Bantam Books.

limiting thought patterns that obscure your ability to recognize and connect with this innate empowerment. You are already your Higher Self when you are focusing on what you are doing, coming from your heart, or receiving creative insights. Through awareness and learning to trust in your Higher Self, your innate intelligence and wisdom will be revealed.

Your Higher Self is your connection to the essence of both your inner and outer beauty. Its manifestation is inclined to attainment - both spiritual and physical. As you open up and begin to trust in the intelligent wisdom of your Higher Self you will expand your ability to attain weight loss and vitality, and in the process discover that .....**everything serves a purpose.**

....Everything Serves a Purpose

There are two essential aspects to losing weight. The first, which has already been dealt with, is understanding how you create yourself overweight: how you mentally, emotionally, physically and spiritually give form to your inclination. The second, concerns discovering how being overweight serves you - the intention behind the form. In other words, besides the fact that being overweight is symptomatic of overeating, what inner intention is it fulfilling? In your need to restore balance, what unattended to psychological issue manifests as overweight?

Everything serves a need and a purpose; every relationship, every situation, every choice you make.....even being overweight serves you in a very necessary way. Every aspect of your life fulfils the intention of helping you to regain balance, liberation and fulfilment. Yes, everything serves the necessary purpose of leading you forward to where you need to be in order to further your development and growth. This embraces not only your physical, but also your spiritual progress.

It is not so much that people and situations outside of you are the problem, but rather that people and situations act to mirror that which you need to look at. When you dislike someone, or something, you are experiencing your inner self. Your responses reflect that which is within you.

If objects were not able to reflect light, you would not be able to see them. As a voyager in outer space you would be in total darkness if there were no planetary bodies to reflect the light of stars. The world of physicality affords us the opportunity of observing those personal issues that are not always apparent.

Overweight reveals in a physical form that which we are not dealing with at an emotional level. Much as overweight discloses that which we have missed, so too guilt, anger, fear, and violence reveal that which is hidden within us. Everything is either symptomatic, or symbolic of our inclination. If this were not so, we would not be able to discover and fulfil our purpose!

There is nothing that happens in your life that does not serve this principle. Once you begin to see this connection, you begin to value life's instruction - you also begin to see the broader pattern and purpose to the events that touch you. Jung talked of *syncronicity* - meaningful coincidence. Nothing happens by chance - nothing is insignificant. The circumstances and incidents you experience - all these things are significant and necessary for your growth and development - everything is connected to your future. The problem arises when you fail to see these connections - when you miss the opportunity to appreciate that everything serves a purpose.

Awarded the Best Actress award at the Montreal Film Festival and lauded for her performance as the battered Maori wife who finds the strength and courage to stand up to her brutal husband in the film, "Once Were Warriors", Rena Owen's life story unfolds in a series of meaningful coincidences that reveals a pattern as startling as the narrative of the film.

Born in New Zealand to an English mother and Maori father, Rena found herself in a social milieu where there was very little prospect for self-advancement. From an early age Rena had an urge to creatively express herself. Unsure of how to fulfil this urge and with no other Maori role models to emulate, she began dancing and singing with a Maori cultural group. Her interest in music and fashion led her as a young woman to travel to England where she became involved in the punk scene. This inevitably led to drugs and a stint in jail. Interviewed about her life, Rena intimates that being caught and imprisoned afforded her the opportunity to deal with her dependency and re-evaluate her life.[24] One of the decisions she made on being released was to fulfil her creative need to express herself - to become an actress.

Desperate for work, Rena happened one day to be shown an ad in a magazine calling for actresses from New Zealand. She duly answered the ad. During her interview she sensed that her lack of experience would not get her the part. On impulse she asked what the play was about. The play happened to be about seven women that were serving time in prison, so she got the part. This enabled Rena to develop her acting

---

[24] Article: From Heroin to Heroine by Barry Ronge in The Star January 6, 1995

ability and qualify for an Equity card. No sooner had the play finished than the next coincidence occurred. She was trying to learn how to meditate when she came across the telephone number of an organization that taught Transcendental Meditation. So Rena duly phoned up. A misdialed number resulted in her contacting an organization called Clean Break. The organization was a theatre company that employed only ex-prisoners. The consequence of this was an acting career that took her around Canada and Europe.

Finally after completing a stint with Clean Break, Rena returned home to discover that Maori's were no longer discriminated against and that it was possible for her to find work in theatre and film. Some time after her arrival back she was sent the script for, "Once Were Warriors". With shocked astonishment Rena realized that the role of Beth, a young woman married to a violent man who finally finds the strength and courage to leave her husband and regain her dignity as a Maori woman was a role that could have been written for her. Her life experiences in some inevitable way had been preparing her for this demanding character part. Rena's role in this low budget film that involved many of the other parts being filled by people that had never acted before, has been artistically and commercially acclaimed in film festivals around the world.

Rena's story is an illustration of synchronicity, and how .....*everything serves a purpose*. Your life, in it's own distinct way is determined by the same principles. Your talents, abilities, and experiences are of necessity unique to your particular situation and purpose, however it unfolds. In the patterning of these experiences lies the meaning.

Meaning is derived by the way in which you view your personal experiences. Generally we are inclined to evaluate in terms of 'success' or 'failure'. But there is another way of viewing personal matters that goes beyond the censure of either 'success' or 'failure'.

Chapter Four

Beyond Success or Failure

One of the recurring and central themes throughout this book is the principle of the whole, the concept of unity and Oneness - the moving beyond the limitations of right or wrong, good or bad, acceptance or rejection, success or failure. What is fundamental in attempting to grasp this notion, is that any form of judgement restricts your ability to attain fulfilment. When you begin to view matters from a position of centredness, from a recognition that beneath and beyond all self-judgement lies an essence that is whole and undivided, you begin the process of actuating your full potential. The qualities of harmony, equilibrium and fulfilment are attributes of this state. When we talk of being whole, we are referring to the fact that it is not only possible, but it is the sole purpose and function of your entire being to incline to the manifestation of this unaffected state.

The way in which you view yourself determines your ability to bring about and sustain personal change. Inevitably, your ability to lose weight is determined by this viewpoint. If you can begin to shed the concept of having to always think in terms of right or wrong, success or failure, or any other polar opposite, you can entertain a way of looking at matters that is so much broader and more inclusive.

The recognition of the dynamic interplay between extremes is articulated in the writings of the Greek philosopher Heraclitus of Ephesus in 6 BCE. Heraclitus perceived the universe to be in a process of continual change and movement; and, out of this continuum emanated the dynamic interaction of opposites. Heraclitus defined any pair of opposites as a whole.

Consciousness is by its very nature divisive; it separates everything into opposites. It creates dichotomies of right and wrong, good and bad, success and failure, you and I, high and low, dark and light. In fact these divisions run through every strata of our existence. We even define ourselves in terms of inner and outer, conscious and unconscious, fat and thin ..... the personal polarities are interminable.

This tendency to separate begins with birth, which is in itself a physical separation from our mothers womb, and ends with the final polarity of death. At another level, the birth of the ego embodies our spiritual separation from the Source. Behind this polarity lies a singularity that is referred to by many esoteric teachings as Oneness, Beingness, or the All.

The relationship between polarity and the whole is embedded in the very form and essence of nature. The tides of the ocean are determined by the cadence of the ebb and flow of the sea. Without the tidal ebb there would be no flow. The ocean exists because of these polarities. At a fundamental level the cycles and rhythms of life are defined by the polarities of hot and cold, day and night, summer and winter, the waxing and waning of the moon, and all the other movements that constitute the full spectrum of earthly life. For every type of matter there exists antimatter with opposite, but equal properties; for every electron there exists a positron; and for every particle there exists an antiparticle. At all levels of existence the interdependency between polarities indicates that behind this separation exists a singularity of purpose.

"....There is, however, an underlying, more inward pattern and what we observe as this tendency in nature towards equilibrium is underlain by the extended causality of the One within the many. It is part of the way in which the polarity of opposites or the world of duality is manifested." [1]

Physics has a wonderful way of demonstrating that polarities underlie the whole through the principal of complementarity. The concept of complementarity explains the paradox of the wave-particle duality in light. Light contains both waves and particles. As we know from rudimentary school physics, a wave can't be a particle (for waves are frequencies), and a particle can't be a wave.

Experimentally you can view light as either a wave-like, or particle-like aspect, but not as both. Waves and particles are mutually exclusive, or complementary aspects of light. You can't view both aspects of light at the same time. Yet light contains both aspects! Both are necessary in order to understand light.

In the field of quantum mechanics the wave-particle duality signalled the termination of viewing the world in terms of polarities of **either-or**. Quantum theory inclusively embraces the fact that something can be both **this** and **that** - a wave and a particle, and that in order to form a complete picture both aspects are necessary. As the ebb and flow of the tides form the integrated expression of the ocean, or, as the push and pull of gravity holds the solar

---

[1] *The Secret of the Creative Vacuum:Man and the Energy Dance* by John Davidson published by C.W.Daniel Company Ltd.

system together, so too **Fat** and **Thin** constitute the integrated expression of your underlying wholeness. The Buddhist Mahayana philosopher Nagarjuna writing in the first century C.E. declares: *"Things derive their beauty and nature by mutual dependence and are nothing in themselves."*

Polarity is our means of touching and reconnecting with the whole. The world of polarity leads us to inevitably consider movement away from the extremes of personal judgement towards the centre of understanding and self-acceptance.

The tendency to continually judge yourself in terms of 'fat' or 'thin', only acts to limit your ability to direct your life. The self-criticism that cyclically draws you into its energy depleting vortex, only serves to perpetuate overeating and imbalance. Hating food or your body, or thinking in terms of success or failure, or indulging in any other form of polarity only reinforces conflict.

"Goodness is no better than evil, pleasure is no better than pain and light is no better than darkness, for they are all the gifts of the Creator. They all play vital and necessary roles in the school of evolution called Earth."[2]

At every level polarity pervades our existence. The interdependency between polar opposites indicates that behind separation, exists a singularity of purpose. These polarities are neither good nor bad, right nor wrong....they merely form parts of the whole. They enable us to find the centre and begin restoring the balance that is so necessary for personal fulfilment.

---

[2] *The Vision of Ramala* by published by The C.W.Daniel & Company Ltd.

....About Restoring Balance

".....nature works continually to restore us to the ideal weight, stature, health, efficiency and everything else, when we remove the obstacles in the way of her remarkable healing power."[3]

Losing weight is about restoring balance in your life. *Over-weight, dis-ease* or any other physical *imbalance* is an attempt at *re-creating* balance in your life. The body in itself can never be said to be ill or imbalanced for the body merely acts as the receiver of the messages that the mental body puts out. As a highly sensitive organism these messages resonate through the body. The persistence of these messages determines their amplification.

Issues, both mental and emotional that you fail to address in your life are stored away in the memory of your subconscious mind. They do not simply fade away because you have conveniently forgotten them. They continue to shadow you wherever you go. The longer they are left unaddressed, the more they grow. And, this is where your holistic body is so smart. In it's attempt to make you aware of what you are not attending to and re-create balance, it whispers to you. It sends you messages of what you are not heeding in the form of feelings, ideas, hopes, dreams, whims and fantasies. The messages it sends you are of a subtle nature. They do not necessarily hit you on the head! But, if you continue to ignore the whispers of your innate intelligence, if the message is lost, your consciousness is forced to manifest the in-

---

[3] *Food Combining for Health* by Doris Grant and Jean Joice published by Thorsons.

tention in a more visible and tangible form - through physical manifestation.

Everything serves a purpose - and the purpose of overweight is to make you aware of that which you are not heeding at an inner level. The longer you ignore the message, the greater the physical manifestation. If neglected, as in the case of overweight, your health can be affected resulting in illness, or in some cases ultimately even in death.

In the manifestation of overweight is the intention of what you have attempted to deny.

Much like your car, the fact that you ignore an unusual noise in the engine does not necessarily mean that the noise will go away. The noise which is the result of something obviously wrong will continue. The longer you ignore it the more damage it will create. From the unattended issue will come a crack in the engine mounting, which if still disregarded will cause the mounting to snap off. This will now place stress on the other engine mountings. The logical consequence of this, is that if left unaddressed, your engine will eventually fall out of the chassis.

As the body can never be said to be the cause of overweight, so too it is important that you do not now see the mind as the cause of any imbalance in your life. For neither the body nor the mind is ever imbalanced or ill - it is only the *thoughts you think* that cause you to move out of the moment and into the world of polarity. Imbalance and illness does not originate in the mind, but rather through the mind.

The divisions of mind and body merely allow us to understand the different functions, they do not imply that they are in any way separate. Mind and body are inextricably linked together to form the whole, and only through the division of thought do we identify and create separation.

In principle the body/mind is a homeostatic organism; that is, it demands that balance be maintained for it to function effectively. The holistic body is endowed naturally to restore balance at all levels. The hypothalamus is a crucial part of the brain and is responsible for the maintenance of homeostasis. It is involved not only in regulating the bodily functions of temperature, the monitoring of the blood, hunger and the like, but it is also the organ that controls sleep, emotions and sexual behaviour. These homeostatic inclinations of the physical body constantly restore balance to maintain an optimum state of health. Every aspect of the human make-up displays the attempt by the holistic body to retain or if necessary regain the natural and fulfilling state of balance. At all levels your entire being is inclined to the maintenance of a state of balance.

"Generally speaking, when one or more factors or constraints are applied or added to any energy system, it is characteristic of nature's processes to attempt to include the new factors within the existing equilibrium. When, however, the new factors or input energy push the system beyond the point at which the old kind of equilibrium can be maintained, then - rather than becoming chaotic - nature transforms or reorganizes herself into a different state of equilibrium. Nature has an in-built preference for order and equilibrium, everything is arranged that way."[4]

This principle of balance applies equally to that of our consciousness. At a consciousness level

---

[4] *The Secret of the Creative Vacuum: Man and the Energy Dance* by John Davidson published by C.W.Daniel & Co. Ltd.

those issues that we do not complete or resolve are eventually compelled to manifest physically and in so doing restore a form of balance.

Through the physical manifestation the symptom restores balance.

Whatever we deny at a consciousness level we live out in the symptom. Let us say, for example, you have failed to deal with a past trauma. If, as a recurring pattern, you fail to address this, it will eventually manifest in a physical form, either as overweight or some other physical condition. The sole purpose of being overweight or illness is to make you whole. The body is the means by which the psyche can in a tangible and obvious way indicate to you that which needs attending to.

Imbalance arises out of those issues that we do not address. Polarities force us to either accept or reject. What we accept we deal with and integrate into our life and what we reject we push aside. It is these denied aspects that form our *shadows*. These shadows do not simply disappear because we are seemingly unaware of them. They lodge themselves in our subconscious mind where they insidiously grow. If denied for long enough they come back manifesting physically as overweight, illness, or other forms of imbalance. In the holistic body's attempt to restore balance the issue that has not been addressed manifests in the form of a symptom and in so doing recreates a form of balance. It is important to recognize that even though this form of balance may be disagreeable - it is a means of dealing with the unattended issue.

One of the reasons why dieting does not permanently resolve the issue of overweight is because the underlying cause has not been dealt with. Sure you can lose weight through following a diet but you will only be able to maintain this through the perpetual suppression of your desires; for the unaddressed issue will continue to recur in one form or another. The fact that you cauterize the wart on your finger does not mean that you have removed the root cause. The wart will simply grow back or reappear somewhere else on your body. Only once you have dealt with the source of the issue are you able to effectively resolve the symptom.

The other aspect to your shadows is that they can take on any form; they do not necessarily manifest in the same way each time. If for example, you continued dieting indefinitely, you would obviously not put on unwanted weight, but because you have not dealt with the denied issue it will manifest in some other form. It will manifest as illness or some other condition of physical imbalance. The intention of what has not been addressed in your life will keep on coming back. Each time the manifestation will become more and more obvious and increase in severity.

How you observe your shadows determines how effectively you restore balance. As the authors Thornwald Dethlefsen and Rudiger Dahlke MD in their book *The Healing Power of Illness* point out: there are two primary approaches that you can follow in your attempt to find the significance behind the symptom. The first of these is that of trying to establish the line of cause; the other is that of being able to discover meaning through an awareness of the underlying pattern to your behaviour (in this case overeating).

Attempting to determine the cause of why you are overweight necessitates that you take a causal approach. Causality is based on the principle of cause and effect, and is grounded in the logic of left brain hemisphere thinking. In its analytical approach it requires that you are able to establish a chain of events, a sequence of justifications. Let us say for example you recognize that you started to put on weight at the age of fifteen. You are able to recognize that the cause of this was because you felt insecure. Your insecurity in turn was caused by the fact that you were failing your grades. This was caused by the fact that you had a bad relationship with your father. The reason you had a bad relationship with your father was because you felt your father neglected to take an interest in you. The reason your father neglected to take an interest in you was caused by the resentment he felt towards you because he felt your mother attempted to compensate in the relationship by giving you attention that your father felt he should be receiving ....and so the line of causality interminably continues. As you can clearly see, the chain of causes is endless. At what point do you stop this line of reasoning? Which of these causes is the primary cause for compulsion to overeat? This sequential aspect of causality makes you aware of horizontal relationships, it places you in the past, rather than the present. Causality of necessity, places the cause as something outside of you. It is as if by finding a cause you can blame something outside of yourself as having created you overweight.

The other way of viewing imbalance is through the analogical thinking of the right brain hemisphere. Whereas the left hemisphere excels in logical sequences the right hemisphere thinks in images. It is this ability to think in images that gives the right hemisphere the benefit of being able to recognize *patterns*. And it is in the patterns of behaviour that *meaning* can be found. You will be able to recognize that either fear, anxiety, frustration or the like, underlie the pattern to your overeating.

Experiments conducted with split-brain patients reveal that if pieces of a shape are felt with the left hand (the right brain controls the left side of the body), the patient is able to associate the pieces with the whole shape. This same ability is decidedly limited if the other hand is used. You are able to recognize someone you know instantly in a crowd through your right hemisphere functions; whereas, if you were to rely on your left hemisphere, you would have to go through the sequential function of isolating and identifying each separate feature and comparing each of these to each person in the crowd. Not only does your left hemisphere operate on the basis of separation and comparison, it would not be able to recognize the person if for example, they changed their hair colour. On the other hand, right hemisphere analogy enables you to see the whole rather than merely the parts that make up the whole. The right hemisphere is able to make these assessments accurately and instantaneously.

Analogy enables you to relate things to each other by determining the underlying pattern that exists between different forms. Identifying the pattern to the behaviour that surrounds your need to overeat, your recurrent attacks of flu, or headaches, enables you to discover the inner meaning to the symptom. It may be fear, anger, unrequited love, or any other unattended to emotion that has caused you to find fulfilment through overeating. If you are able to honestly look at the symptom, in this case overweight, and in the process discover the meaning, you discover something about yourself. It is this process that assures personal growth. In this, is the movement of liberation and the attainment of balance and weight loss.

To be able to understand the meaning to the symptom there is no need to go back into the past. Whatever you see there is merely the same shadow in a different guise. For shadows can manifest in any form. They are of a capricious and variable nature. For example, lack of self-love can manifest as aggression or withdrawal, or as overweight or underweight. Over time the same shadow repeats itself in various ways. All that is required is that you become aware of the pattern. Within the pattern lies the meaning to that which you have failed to address.

Having reached the point where you are able to now recognize the meaning to your need to overeat, the question arises: What to do? Normally, one would attempt to suppress or change what one sees. Any attempt to either censor or suppress the aspect that is being denied will only force it back into darkness. Judgement of any form, whether it be right or wrong, good or bad, draws your attention away from the issue and recreates conflict.

Awareness is the centre between judgement, between right or wrong, suppression or declaration. Awareness is the means of shining light onto your shadows. Observing without judgement, without prejudice, gives back the power to your centre. Shadows only exist in darkness. Once they are exposed, their power fades away.

Overweight or illness are all signs that are pointing to what you have failed to integrate at a consciousness-level. As hunger is symptomatic of a need, so over-eating is symptomatic of an attempt to find balance. In the symptom, in the physical form of overweight or illness lies the means for addressing your most veiled issues.

The need for balance in our lives is confirmation that everything serves a purpose. Whatever we experience offers us the potential to expand our advancement.

Overweight offers you the invaluable opportunity to see that which you have difficulty in perceiving at a consciousness-level. In a physical form you are presented with the wonderful opportunity of seeing something that may not be that obvious. Without a TV screen you would not be able to see the television waves that carry the images. And, without the manifestation of overweight, you would possibly not be aware of that which you have psychologically failed to address.

"In reality all human endeavour serves but one aim: learn to see the connections more clearly ("to become more aware" as we say) - not thought to alter things. There is, after all, nothing whatever to alter or improve - apart from one's own way of seeing."[5]

You do not necessarily arrive at meaning through analysis, rather, by being able to see in the patterns of your behaviour the underlying meaning, you arrive at a deeper substantive understanding of issues. This process enables you to discover the underlying intention to your eating behaviour. Every time you are driven to overeat or binge, you will begin to see the intention of this as a feeling - a feeling of failure, fear, anxiety, frustration, self-rejection, insecurity, a need for fulfilment, or some other form

---

[5] *The Healing Power of Illness* by Thornwald Dethlefsen and Rudiger Dahlke M.D. published by Element Books.

of repressed emotion. As Louise L.Hay points out in her book *Heal Your Body - The Mental Causes of Physical Illness and the Metaphysical Way to Overcome Them*: Whatever you physically manifest will reflect that which you are not attending to. Louise Hay sites some of the psychological causes for overweight as insecurity, hidden anger and self-rejection. For example: excess fat carried around the hips would be an indication of holding anger towards one's parents. Weight carried on the thighs is related to anger that stems from childhood. Excess weight carried around the mid-rift area suggests being denied nourishment.

Remember, the means to identifying that which you are not attending to at a psychological level, is in the pattern. Before moving onto the next section it is important that you give some time and attention to the following questions:

In what way does being overweight serve you?

....

....

....

....

The next time you feel an irrepressible urge to go on an eating spree, be aware of your thoughts. Take note of your thought pictures. Put down how you 'represent' these pictures i.e. are your pictures large or small, bright or dark etc.?

....

....

....

....

Try to recognise the emotional responses that accompany this need to overeat. Write these down.

....

....

....

Take note of how you physically 'represent' when you have the urge to overeat. Write down what you observed. Be as detailed as possible.

....

....

....

....

What did you learn about yourself and your need to overeat?

....

....

....

Chapter Five

The Beauty of Self

A fundamental necessity in any process of transformation is the establishment of a set of conditions that support your actions. These conducive conditions uphold you in your quest for attainment - they establish the matrix for growth and change.

In order for any living organism to optimally grow and flourish, conditions that nurture are required. For a seed to grow, bud and flower, right climate and nourishment are necessary. So too, personal growth and change can only take root in an intimate setting that is supportive and nurturing of transformative change. It is very difficult to lose weight if you have a negative self-image, if you are unable to elicit affirmative self-beliefs, and are incapable of assuming responsibility for your choices.

Discovering the power of self embodies the realization of your innate beauty. This process contains the acknowledgement that what you think, feel, and believe, is what you inevitably manifest.

The self embodies multidimensional potentiality. Within this capacity, the dimensions of Self-Love, Self-Belief, and Self-Responsibility sustain the visage
of self. The first of these - the dimension of Self-Love forms one of the fundamental pillars of support that is central to the attainment of weight loss.

Self-Love

As you are is all you need to be! This is not a statement of flattery or a summation of myopic self analysis; rather it is an acknowledgement and acceptance of who you are. It is an acknowledgement that you are unique, attractive, vital, imaginative, unlimited, loving, and much more than can ever be listed here. This acknowledgement also embodies the recognition that personal development is an ongoing process; and that in order to connect with the whole you need to move beyond any form of self limiting judgement.

Love of self does not imply an egoistic, smug attitude, but implies rather a deep abiding acceptance of who you are. It contains an awareness of your unlimited capacity and potential to be. It is an acknowledgement of all that has brought you to this point in time.

It is difficult to imagine being able to even think about losing weight while you dislike yourself, or your body. In this state you can only think of punishing and denying yourself - repeating the same old limiting beliefs and eating patterns that caused you to put on weight in the first place. But, turn this around through a deep love of all that you are, and losing weight and self-attainment become self-fulfilling enactments. Love of self also means acknowledging your ability to manifest. As you are right now is proof of this. Self-love embodies not only your outer beauty but also your inner beauty; your ability to care, love, laugh, and all the other expressions that make you a whole being.

Until you learn to truly love yourself (that includes your body as it is now), you will never be able to effortlessly effect the changes you want. You may temporarily accomplish thinness through deprivation and discipline, but this state can only be sustained through the imposition of will-power and self-denial. Will-power contains suggestions of struggle and denial, it demands effort. It is incapable of self perpetuation.

Hating yourself, or your body, implies that you hold a limiting self-perception. How can you lose weight while you hold a negative image of yourself? Losing weight is an affirmative energy - being critical a negative energy! They are two opposing energies. When you are able to truly love yourself as you are now, then you can direct change from an empowered position. These perceptions and feelings will release energy. This release of energy will assist you in the changes you wish to make: losing weight no longer becomes such a disaffected process. The more you learn to love yourself, the quicker your body will respond, and the more beautiful and healthy your body will be.

When you judge yourself, you are in effect saying that you are no more than what you appear to be: what you see is what you are! You are not acknowledging both your inner and outer potential. When you say to yourself, "I hate my body", or, "I can never be slim", you are declaring that you are a limited physical entity. You are denying the full promise of your being. On the other hand, when you recognize your potentiality, you acknowledge that your dimensionality enfolds the boundless endowment of your mental, emotional, physical and spiritual aspects.

It seems that often our self-esteem is determined by how we compare to others, or how we think others see us. Through this type of reflective judgement we arrive at an assessment of ourselves. We often do not appreciate that self-esteem is in fact a self regard and a respect; a love of what is, rather than what is not. Comparison is an exclusive process - it excludes rather than includes. It is a limited perspective. When you compare yourself to someone else you are not including the *big picture* of what you are; and you are most definitely not simply just a face, a pair of legs, or just a body! You are a spiritual, emotional, mental and physical entity. And, as you are beginning to realize, these expressions have unlimited potential - this is the *big picture*. So why choose to define yourself by accepting a limiting outlook. Learn to acknowledge your potential as well as your attributes. We all have our own special qualities and we are all created equal.

As long as you compare yourself to others you will be caught in the realm of judgement. These thoughts act as a negative energy and dissipate your power to attain. It is important to begin becoming aware of how you sit in judgement of yourself. Often your self-image is constructed through a process of comparison. Learn to become aware of this in your daily activities and interactions. When you catch yourself judgementally evaluating yourself, do not criticise or try to stop yourself in the process. Simply watch as though you were an impartial observer.

You will notice that by simply being aware of your thoughts, that the power of these judgemental thoughts dissipates. Holding these thoughts up to the light of observation causes them to lose their power. If you try to suppress or deny your thoughts, you are judging yourself once again. The mind is a master at deception. There is only one way to escape the cyclical pattern of self-judgement, and that is by simply becoming aware. Awareness releases the energy that you require for a deeper understanding and appreciation of yourself. Bhagwan Shree Rajneesh has this to say about being unique:

"To carry the idea of comparison you are carrying the seeds of illness which will create misery and nothing else. Comparison creates hell. Heaven is an inner space where you live a life uncompared. You simply live yourself, it is your life, you are you - just think of the beauty of it, the tremendous purity of it.

....Just think ....the whole world disappears and you alone are left. God takes away the whole world and only you are left, nobody else. Then what will you be - strong, weak , intelligent, unintelligent, beautiful, ugly?

Then who will you be? All comparisons disappear, you will simply be yourself. That is the way to be.

....Just think of it this way: God has never created anybody else like you and he will never create anybody else like you. God has created only one you - only one you, mind - and he is never going to repeat you again. This is your uniqueness. Feel grateful, feel thankful. Once you start comparing you feel ungrateful. Why has he created somebody more beautiful than you, or somebody more intelligent than you? You are bringing misery upon yourself. He has created only you, he has conferred uniqueness on you. It is a gift. Uniqueness is a gift of God."[1]

---

[1] *Tao The Pathless Path* by Bhagwan Shree Rajneesh, published by Rajneesh Foundation.

If you wish to compete, then compare. Standards require comparative measures; which is fine if you are an athlete, an engineer, or a manufacturer; but as a unique, dynamic human being what is going to form the basis to your standards, and who are you competing against? What would form the basis to your standard of physical beauty? Is beauty not an all-embracing thing! For beauty is not just the outer, but the inner too. As in nature, beauty takes on multifarious forms and hues - there is no ultimate form of beauty. If you really need to compare, then compare yourself to your unlimited potential. Acknowledge your individuality and realise that it is not necessary to compete, only to grow. Personal growth requires no critical comparison, for whatever stage you are at in your life, is all that is necessary for your development at that point in time. Personal growth and expansion are the building blocks of your future, for it is only through facing issues that you expand your potential, and in this comes the liberation of self-love and acknowledgement. Personal growth is not a linear process that you measure against someone else, but rather a dynamic multi-dimensional continuance of self. Personal growth ensures a commensurate love of self.

Certainly we can't deny that we all see ourselves as being different to each other. The way in which we view this difference is the difference between *identification* and *comparison*. Identification is our ability to define ourselves.

Identification is an inclusive acknowedgement that you are part of something more expansive than just yourself. When you identify with something you are taking note of its qualities; you are not critically judging the differences. Identification is an awareness that contains within it the inclusion that we are all uniquely different. If you can begin to acknowledge the creative principle of turning within, reflecting on your inner beauty, then you can drop your continual outward comparisons and begin to nourish your love of self. You can most certainly acknowledge others for their beauty, attainment or any other quality that you recognize, but this should not be a process of personal denigration.

Learning to love yourself means accepting yourself as you are now. Acceptance does not imply that you do not have choice, in fact acceptance grants you choice. It is an enabling state that permits you to draw on your personal resources. On the other hand, self-denial implies that your choices are rather limited. If you are unable to love yourself being overweight, then you only have one choice - and that is to lose weight in order to love yourself. If you are unable to do this - then you are unable to accept yourself. If you can't accept yourself then you either drop into a state of depression, or immerse yourself in some other form of excessive behavior. On the other hand, if you accept the way you are, if you love yourself, then within this acknowledgment you are empowered to direct change. You are presented with choices that range beyond the limitations of self denial.

Learning to develop self-love begins by getting in touch with all the wonderful qualities and attributes you have. By acknowledging yourself you implant a recognition of your full potential. Affirm your beauty and being by doing the following exercise:

Write down all your good points. Begin with your physical attributes; start at the top and move down your body. List everything you like about yourself. If you have beautiful lustrous hair, put this down. If your eyes are your strong feature, or you like the shape of your calves, list this. Put down every detail that you feel you like about yourself:

....

....

....

....

....

Write down all your capabilities. Any skills, sporting abilities, artistic abilities, or any other talents that you may have:

....

....

....

....

....

Make a list of everything you have been a success at. This includes what you achieved when you were at school, university, work, your relationships. Include all areas of your life. As you think of more things keep adding to your list.

....

....

....

....

....

Once you have completed this, write down all your endearing emotional capacities. This includes your capacity to feel compassion for others, your ability to care for family and friends, your love of nature and animals.

....

....

....

....

Now write down all the ways you can show self-appreciation. Put down the ways in which you can reward yourself for all that you are. If your idea of pleasure is a massage, or an exotic holiday in the Caribbeans, put it down. Whatever brings you pleasure and fulfilment - your rewards can be anything, small or large.

....

....

....

....

Now begin acknowledging yourself by doing these things. Enact the smaller things on a daily basis, and plan the larger things for the future. Make a resolution to start finding time to appreciate yourself.

What self-affirmation are you going to remember to say to yourself over the next few weeks?

....

....

Review

Read over all your attributes as often as you can. Get a new sense of yourself: see and feel your beauty. The stronger your feelings, the sooner you will begin to manifest this new awareness. Through loving yourself you endorse your capacity for fulfilment and the enactment of your potentiality.

Take your list of attributes and attach it to some prominent spot either on your cupboard, or fridge door. Read over your list as often as you can, reinforce this affirmative image of yourself. Repetition is one of the powerful tools of the mind. Repetition reprograms your subconscious mind to enact your positive strategies. Bear in mind that you have created yourself as you are today through the repetition of certain recurring thought patterns. These dominant thought patterns, or core beliefs accrete to form the second dimension of potentiality - the dimension of Self-Belief.

Self-Belief

One of the most encouraging and inspirational stories that I have come across is that of a woman who was diagnosed as having cancer of the vagina. Despite her doctors pleas, she had the belief and the conviction to forgo surgery and heal herself. Barely six months later an astounded medical profession were compelled to concede that she had tested clear of any form of cancer. But for an indomitable belief in her innate capacity to self heal, this astonishing incident would not have taken place. The woman concerned was none other than Louise L. Hay, the authoress of *Heal Your Body*.

What enables those individuals that against all odds are able to achieve the seemingly impossible? One quality must surely be the attribute of self-belief. The ability to overcome and face personal adversity is only possible if you are able to direct your state of mind - if your are able to believe in Self.

Belief is the substance of your reality. What you believe, ultimately determines your outcome. If you believe that you will fail, then you will most surely fail. If you believe in your innate empowerment then no obstacle will impede your capacity to lose weight, heal yourself or swim the deepest sea. Beliefs enable you to have a vision of what you *deserve*, They give you the thrust to reach out and claim that which is rightfully yours.

Throughout history, beliefs have enabled people to create their realities. Gandhi's deep belief in non-violent transformation enabled him to unite his people in a way that was inconceivable. Nelson Mandela's unshakeable belief in the emancipation of his people enabled him to endure twenty seven years of incarceration. The early Christians believed so deeply in their faith that their persecution did not deter them from spreading the word of Christ. All the great social and religious movements of our time have been fuelled by the deep conviction of belief.

Beliefs can either be the most enabling states you can create, or they can be the most limiting. In fact the power of belief is so powerful that in some tribal societies the mere accusation of a sorcerer can cause death. Medical studies on the placebo effect also clearly indicate the power of belief. In double blind tests patients administered placebos recover remarkably from illness even though the fake drugs have no healing power. Medical science is now beginning to advance that brain cells do not necessarily deteriorate with age, but rather deteriorate as a result of belief in the ageing process. Peter Russell in his book, *The Brain Book* states....

"Expectancy and belief are confounding factors in any study of the effects of aging......If people are given to believe that mental potential is going to decrease after twenty, then it is very likely that it will......The human mind is remarkably adept at materializing its own beliefs."[2]

Recently I read an article about a tribe that lives in a remote region of Russia where the average

---

[2] *The Brain Book* by Peter Russell published by Routledge and Kegan Paul.

life span is one hundred and twenty years. The interesting thing about these tribesmen is that they follow no particular diet, and they drink and smoke. After extensive investigation researchers have finally had to conclude that the only reason they can attribute to such longevity, is 'belief'. The people of this particular tribe implicitly believe a normal life span to be about one hundred and fifty odd years.

Beliefs are the conceptual filters that determine our ability to lose weight and attain beauty and health. Our beliefs guide us in the attainment of our dreams and visions. They are potent and energizing forces in our lives.

Self-beliefs can be divided into those beliefs that are socially or collectively determined, and those beliefs that you adopt through personal experience. Both have the power to determine the outcome of your actions.

Collective beliefs reflect social and cultural belief systems that in some way or another colour the way in which we think and act.

The Power of Collective Beliefs

Beyond the Milky Way lie stars of other galaxies; some hundred thousand million different galactic systems are considered to make up the universe. The view we have today of our planet and the universe is quite different to that which astrologers and scientists believed before 1929. In 1929 one of the most important discoveries of the twentieth century was made. The American astronomer Edwin Hubble discovered that the universe is expanding. The notion that the Universe was static had persisted in the minds of men since before Aristotle. This belief was so entrenched in people's minds that even Einstein modified his theory of general relativity to fit the notion of a static universe. In fact this observation was so apparent that astrologers and physicists should have predicted the universe's expansion from Newtons laws of gravity that were formulated in the late 17th century - for if the universe were static it would have contracted under the influence of its own gravity. The paradigm that existed prior to Hubble's seminal discovery eventuated in a limiting framework of thought. This resulted in a widely held belief that hindered science's perception of the universe for hundreds of years.

Paradigms are frameworks of thought; they form the basis to our collective beliefs. Paradigms shape our attitudes, capabilities and potentialities. They are important because they determine what we believe is possible.

In the early 1950s it was believed that it was impossible for man to run the mile in less than four minutes. The four-minute mile presented a barrier to man's psyche. It was only after Roger Banister broke this record in 1954 in a time of 3:59.4 seconds that this psychological barrier was broken. Now that athletes are running the mile routinely under 3:55 seconds it is firmly embedded in man's psyche that this is no longer merely a possibility, but a reality. Because of this new paradigm, this new belief, athletes are running faster times than ever before. At the writing of this book the current record stands at 3:46.32 seconds and I am certain by the time this book is published this record will have been bettered. Man's belief in his ability to achieve has enabled him to continue attaining new earth-shattering records.

Collective beliefs are influential in our lives because we incorporate these ideas at both a conscious and subconscious level. One of the most limiting beliefs that enjoys widespread acceptance and that has determined how we view losing weight, is the belief; 'No pain, no gain'. Another is, 'Nothing comes easy'; without discipline and suffering you can't expect to lose weight or in fact achieve anything of worth. We seem to be wedded to the notion that without tremendous effort and sacrifice significant attainment is not possible. This pervasive belief is so rooted in our minds that our associations of dieting are nearly always attached to emotions like loathing, anxiety, dread, and general reluctance. *There is no natural law that states that 'effort' will necessarily be rewarded!* In fact, it is not *effort*, but being in alignment with your 'holistic' body that brings about substantial personal change. Even in sport this principle is in evidence. For it is not how hard you hit a ball, but how you time your stroke. Additionally, its not how far your ball travels, but how accurate it is!

Another collective belief that severely limits personal growth is that, 'everything takes time'. Here too there is no natural law that states that the passage of time is a necessity, or even an essential requirement for personal change. Personal transformation takes as little, or as much time as you deem necessary. You impose the constraint of time. In fact, were you to make a total and congruent decision with your whole being, you would effect instantaneous change. As already stated in a previous chapter: *Understanding is a state of being that enables one to instantaneously and effortlessly enact knowledge.* Understanding immediately transfers knowledge into action - there is no separation between what you think, feel or do.

In terms of personal growth and development (and this is what losing weight is all about), it is vital that you become aware of the collective beliefs that limit your potential to attain. Awareness of this is the first step to transcending these limitations. By focusing on the acknowledgment that you have all that you need, you can reconfirm your belief in self. The maxim *'gain without pain'*, should form the basis to your new perception of self.

The recognition that we are entering a New Age with renewed possibilities for human development is a new and invigorating paradigm. This emergent realization that we are approaching a period of unusual transformation, and that we are poised to witness major shifts and expanded growth at all levels of personal and global consciousness assists in embedding a new and enabling belief in our potential. This perception is the beginning of a movement back to our essence - back to a unity, a wholeness where everything is connected. Even the line between physics and metaphysics is becoming less distinct every day. The notion of connectedness is moving towards a paradigm, a collective belief of holistic individuation. More than ever before we have the means to reach enabling levels of attainment.

Before proceeding I would like you to write down any collective beliefs that may hinder your ability to lose weight.

....

....

....
....

Spend a few moments reflecting on how you can replace these limiting thought patterns with new enabling collective beliefs. Write these down.

....
....
....
....

The Power of Personal Beliefs

In essence belief is merely a state of mind; an internal representation that evokes a certain behaviour. It is something that you create, based on what you accept, whether it be actual, or merely a proposition. You are not born with certain beliefs. You adopt personal beliefs through experience. You choose what you believe. Your self-beliefs circumscribe what you are capable of achieving. We all have self-beliefs; some of them limiting, and others that enable us to turn potential problems into favourable opportunities.

Self-beliefs are important because they determine how you respond to your food addictions, your body, and all the other situations that touch you. If you believe you are unable to lose weight, then no matter how hard you attempt to face this issue, you will surely fail! On the other hand, belief can be so enabling that even the seemingly impossible is made possible. As a result of an unshakable belief, the Wright brothers gave us air travel.

For something to be held as a belief, it is not necessary that this be a reality. For reality is no different to illusion. Both are determined by what you believe. Both are merely a perception. As stated previously, a belief can be based on either a proposition, or 'reality'. For instance, no one has seen God, yet many believe in God. As a result of this deep belief, many believers are able to face adversity and hardship. Their belief provides the conviction to persevere.

In order to hold a belief, you need to be convinced that it is possible. It need not be a probability, but it certainly must be within the realm of possibility. There is very little that is not possible. Certainly, when it comes to actualizing your self-potential, the possibilities are unlimited. Losing weight is very much a possibility. Once you truly believe in the possibility, the inclination of your mental, emotional, physical and spiritual centres is to realize this intention. The possibility now becomes a very real probability!

Belief permeates many levels of your daily life. If you did not believe that you would arrive safely at your destination, you would certainly not get into your car. Even some of the most cogent arguments about the universe and existence are sometimes inevitably reduced to the realm of belief. Beliefs form the basis to what we experience, whether these experiences be physical, or spiritual.

Beliefs based on past experiences form the core of your future beliefs. By beginning to identify what beliefs hold you back, you hold the means to change these limiting states. There are many different levels of beliefs. There are those beliefs that concern every day matters, and then there are those deeper beliefs that concern your very existence. It is these deep core beliefs that have the most power to affect how you view your potential to attain.

Spend some time examining what beliefs have held you back in the past. Or, another way of looking at the situation is to ask yourself: "What beliefs would I have needed to create myself overweight?" Put these down.

....

....

....

....

One way to create new enabling self-beliefs is to determine what you desire in the future. If you desire to lose 12 pounds (5.5Kg) over a period of three months, then this can form the basis to your new belief. You now believe that it is within your power to attain this weight loss. Remember, thoughts create feelings, and feelings determine what actions you will take in the future. The ability to visualize and experience the feelings of what this will bring you is the key to belief creation.

What new beliefs about yourself would you require to lose weight? Write down those beliefs that would promote weight loss in the future.

....

....

....

....

If you are unequivocal in your belief, then you will manifest the necessary actions to create your intention. You may not necessarily attain this first time round, but you will keep coming back with empowering actions that will establish the conditions necessary for your attainment. One of the finest examples of this is the life story of Abraham Lincoln. Abraham Lincoln, one of the greatest of American presidents tried unsuccessfully for political office from the age of 32 to 59 years of age. It was only in his 60th year that he was elected as president of the United States. His deep rooted self-belief enabled him to finally succeed.

Belief can be summarized as a conviction, a deep sense of your potentiality. Belief is the sanction of your mental, emotional, physical and spiritual empowerment.

So far we have dealt with conscious self-beliefs: those beliefs that are determined by what we consciously think and feel. There is another aspect to personal beliefs that needs considering - and that is the unconscious beliefs we hold.

It is far easier to be aware of your conscious beliefs than your unconscious beliefs. Unconscious beliefs that deny your right to enjoy success and achievement, subvert your assertive actions. On the one hand you may truly see the need to lose weight, and have a sense that you are capable of losing weight, but at the same time unconsciously you may believe that being slim will not serve you. You may for example still be holding onto a negative need to be overweight because it provides you with a feeling and sense of security. It may meet the need of not having to face being attractive, or successful, or any other attribute that will propel you into new areas of experience. The authors Grindler and Bandler mention in their book *Frogs into Princes*, the case of an overweight woman who was able to lose weight, but unable to sustain this weight loss. The problem that this particular woman faced was that when she lost weight she became attractive, and this caused men to be attracted to her. She found it very difficult not to respond to their advances. So, rather than jeopardize her marriage, she put on weight. It was only when she discovered why she was inclined to be overweight and that there other more effective ways of dealing with this issue that she was able to permanently lose weight, which she incidentally was able to do without having to diet. In some cases, fear of succeeding means that you do not have to expose yourself to change. Some people are attached to the 'struggle'. It gives them a feeling of being in control. If things come too easily the person may feel they have lost control to direct their life. Your unconscious limiting beliefs take on many different forms, but they can always be identified by the fact that they are related to fear.

    It is important that you begin to identify these hidden limiting beliefs. By learning to acknowledge your unconscious beliefs you unblock the energy necessary to begin enacting affirmative beliefs.

Exercise

Find a comfortable spot, relax and still your mind. Now go within and ask your Higher Self to assist you in discovering what your hidden limiting beliefs are. Whatever comes up for you write it down. Do not try to understand what is coming up for you, simply write freely and spontaneously. Let it be a release rather than a chore. It doesn't matter whether these beliefs relate to you being overweight, or to some other area of your life. You will eventually begin to see the connectedness. Spend as much time as you need to complete this exercise.

....

....

....

....

At the end of this read over what you have written and see if you can connect these beliefs to your past experiences. See whether they are related to your childhood, your parents or any other life experience. If for example one of your limiting beliefs is; "I can never lose weight", you may connect this to what you heard people say about you in the past. Write this down. Ask yourself now what purpose these beliefs are serving. Try and discover what the payoff is. It may be that you use the fact that you are overweight to justify your situation. Whatever it is, take note of what comes up for you.

....

....

....

....

Now take these limiting beliefs and release them. Acknowledge that they no longer serve your needs: they may have met a need in the past and may have been appropriate for a certain time in your life, but they now no longer serve a need. Thank them, and now focus on assimilating new empowering beliefs.

Affirm that you are beautiful, that the food you eat will support your actions and that by loving yourself more the world will love you more. Affirm your potential to create immeasurably.

As long as you believe that you have to suffer, your life will be filled with pain, hardship, and anguish. The law of attraction states that you will draw to you what you put out. You have the choice to reach out and find joy, succour, and attainment.

And, finally; what new positive beliefs about yourself are you going to bring into your life in the next two days?

....

....

....

....

Self-Responsibility

What, and where you are at this present moment in time, is the sum total of all your past thoughts, beliefs, and actions - both in this life time, and if you believe in reincarnation, in other lifetimes. Through the choices you made, you created yourself overweight, rich, poor, happy, sad, or whatever else you may be. Whether you wish to acknowledge this or not, your situation or condition is a choice. If you are honest and reflect on your life, you must accept that you are responsible for what you created, whether you were conscious or not, of your choices at the time.

If you chose not to recognize that you are responsible for the weight you have gained, or any other situation that you may presently be experiencing, you will not be empowered to change your circumstance.

What you receive in the future, is determined by the choices you make now. And the choices you make now, are in turn dependent on whether or not you are prepared to assume responsibility for what you chose. Self-responsibility involves making choices from a position of being a participator, and not a victim.

If you truly wish to lose weight and direct your life it is imperative that you acknowledge responsibility for the choices you make. Acknowledging responsibility means that you are acknowledging your empowerment. The degree of your achievement will be directly proportionate to the responsibility you assume. Responsibility is also inextricably linked to involvement. Without involvement, without commitment, there is very little chance of sustaining your intentions.

Look at the lives of those that are out there achieving. They would never be where they are today without being totally involved and responsible for what they do. In order to achieve, you need to assume full responsibility for the choices you make, and the actions you take. Achievers are not afraid to risk! The reason they are not afraid to risk is because they accept that they are co-creators in the play of life. Together with the divine gift of life, they are participants in the outcome of their experiences. Whether they initially achieve their intended result or not, they accept responsibility for their choices.

Assuming responsibility is an acknowledgement of your empowerment - it is a validation of your freedom of will and your right to choose.

The more you assume responsibility for your choices, the greater your achievements will be. There is also the attendant inference that by accepting responsibility, you exercise your choice from a completely different position. You now realize that every outcome has a bearing on your life, and you make choices with deliberation. Self-responsibility is one of the important underlying denominators to attainment.

Accepting responsibility for your body as it is, is an important step in your progress towards losing weight. Instead of blaming circumstances or others for your predicament, accept that you have control over your life. Accept that what you have chosen in the past may no longer serve your needs; accept that you have the right to choose only that which benefits you. Recognize that you have the power to change your circumstance, and that the choice lies with you.

The foods you eat and the lifestyle you live are matters that *you* determine. It is not the food, alcohol, or cigarettes that have the power - you have the power, you have the power of choice. Ruth White in her book *Working with your Chakras*, sums up empowerment wonderfully. She states; *"Power is a principle, and empowerment is the process of making use of that principle."* Additionally, *choice* is a principle, and empowerment is the process of making use of that principle.

If you give food your power then recognize this as a choice you have made. Accept responsibility. You will discover that when you start making choices from a position of accountability that you will begin to feel and act differently. You will gain a renewed sense of self and begin to make choices that serve you. The sooner you begin to accept responsibility for the choices you make, the sooner you will lose weight.

Accept the responsibility that it is your birthright to be slim, beautiful, healthy, happy, and fulfilled in every area of your life. Self-responsibility is part of the process of transformation; it is a measure of your personal development and power. Before moving onto the next section, spend a few minutes reflecting on the following exercise:

How can acknowledging self-responsibility help you to lose weight ?

....

....

....

> ## *The Choice Loop!*
> *Remember, what you receive in the future is determined by the choices you make. And the choices you make, are in turn dependent on whether or not you are prepared to assume responsibility for what you choose.*

Chapter Six

Power Tools

As with all personal and creative areas, the use of specific tools facilitates your quest for attainment. The previous chapters have been primarily concerned with understanding and directing your innate empowerment. This section presents you with the means to draw on some of your additional resources - your **power tools**. These tools enable you to give impetus and direction to losing weight. They assist in focusing the energy and forces that shape your outcome.

The first of these power tools is the source to all your dreams and visions - 'the pouring in of ideas and feelings'.

Inspiration

Have you ever wondered how a Leonardo da Vinci, a Michelangelo, a Picasso, a Bach, was able to create so awe-inspiringly and so prolifically? Have you ever pondered what the source to their creativity was?

All creativity is sparked by inspiration. Inspiration is variously described as; *the arousal by, or as if by supernatural or divine influence; the infusion of ideas and feelings; the act of breathing in.*

It is interesting to note that the word *infuse*, is derived from the Latin word *functure*, which means 'to pour into'. Inspiration can therefore be taken literally as 'the pouring in of ideas and feelings'. Alternatively, inspiration is associated with, 'breathing in'. Breath in metaphysical terms, and for that matter even medical terms is related to the giving of life. It is the 'in' breath that initiates life. Not only is inspiration responsible for giving life to your visions and ideas, but it imparts an intensity that enables you to reach out and touch your full potentiality.

Inspiration is that wonderful state that makes you feel that anything is possible. It is the source of your visions, dreams, and aspirations. Without inspiration there is little chance that man would have been able to land on the moon. Inspiration is that part of the creative process where you envisage and experience the colour and magnificence of the plant in bloom, long before you even decide to prepare the soil, or plant the seed.

Whether you wish to attain on a grand scale, or on a more limited scale, you need to be able to draw on inspiration. Before you can even begin to think of losing weight, you need to be inspired. You need to be inspired to create a vision; a vision of beauty, health, and vitality.

We have all experienced that elated feeling when we have been aroused to go out and achieve - where we have dared to go beyond that which we thought was possible. Being inspired is more than merely entertaining an idea, or a thought; inspiration is being elevated to a state where you reach out and glimpse your full potentiality. It is a state that knows no limitations.

Einstein had a vision of the Law of Relativity long before he was able to prove that timespace was curved. It was his inspired vision of beams of light from distant stars bending as they passed celestial bodies like the sun, that motivated him to continue until he was able to validate the principles of relativity. All the great inventors, scientists, writers, and artists have relied on inspiration to create their most elevated and insightful works.

Inspiration knows no boundaries, it is not restricted by analytical thought. In time, it is beyond the past, or present. In consequence, it is beyond measure - it is your most creative state.

Inspiration is essentially a powerful and heady mix of images and emotions. The nature of this state is that it is unqualified. When you are inspired, you do not evaluate whether or not your ideas are necessarily 'realistic', or attainable.

In Chapter Three: Self-Empowerment: The Mental Body, we dealt with how you represent thoughts through images - thought pictures. You did an exercise where you established how you construct your 'enabling' thought pictures. If you now take this strategy of yours and amplify this two to three times - you have an approximation of the measure of 'inspiration'. When you are inspired your images are bigger, your colours brighter. Everything about your picture is intensified and expanded.

Not only are your thoughts more expansive, but your feelings too are more ardent. When you are inspired, you are transported - the intensity of your emotions are elevated. You are directly linked to you heart. There is a strong correspondence between your heart and your head.

One of the definitions used to describe inspiration is; *the arousal by, or as if by supernatural or divine influence*[1]. There is no doubt that when you are stirred and inspired by an idea that there is a

---

[1] The Concise Oxford English Dictionary

strong connective link to your spiritual essence. The sense of one's expansiveness is that its source is of an exalted nature.

When you are 'inspired' you are channelling the combined energies of your spiritual, mental, emotional, and physical bodies.

Exercise

Inspiration is the fount of magnificence. You can be inspired to create a beautiful body and lose weight by daring to dream.

Go within and let your mind relax. Now begin to focus on what you want. Drop your habitual thinking patterns and responses, and imagine how you would look and feel with your new body. Allow your imagination to soar, and at the same time permit yourself to feel your expansiveness. This should be a joyous elevated experience. If need be, use a photo of someone else's body that you admire, or draw on whatever stimulus works best for you.

Now expand the setting of your dream. Imagine all the qualities and benefits that you associate with being firm and slim. It may be acknowledgement, or admiration from others, being able to wear fashionable clothes, feeling confident, enjoying more energy and vitality; whatever it is that is important to you, these are the things to bring to your dream.

As you imagine these things and experience the feelings they arouse, sharpen your images. Enlarge your images as much as you can. Intensify the colour. Instead of hearing mono, hear stereo sound. Increase and intensify all the modalities of your thought picture. Allow your mind to wander. Allow it to transport you to new and invigorating realms where your potential knows no bounds. Allow this process to reveal that which you have denied and hidden through the memories of past experiences.

Now how did that feel? What were the qualities of the feelings you experienced?

....

....

....

....

How does inspiration differ from creative visualization for you?

....

....

....

....

Inspiration is a powerful vision of your capacity to create.

Inspiration contains a sense of what is possible as well as the suggestion of that which is beyond limitation. Due to its emotional intensity, this state is difficult to sustain and is usually of limited duration. But if inspiration can be turned into motivation, then the promise of your dream is within reach. Inspiration is the ground to motivation. Motivation enables you to transform into actuality that which you envisaged in a state of inspiration.

Motivation

Why is it that when you initially decide to embark on something new that you are so motivated, even driven to achieve your visions... but with the passing of time your sense of motivation begins to dissipate and eventually disappears? What at first seemed so easy to do, now becomes harder and harder. Losing weight, going to gym, or giving up smoking become an uphill struggle.

What is motivation, and how do you sustain this state long enough to attain your inspired vision of a slim, healthy body?

Motivation is defined as; *that which incites to action.* In other words, you need to be able to move beyond a state of inspiration to a point where you are able to put into action that which you have envisaged. You need to be able to draw on your inspiration on a continuing basis.

If you are able to discover and record what it is that initially inspires you to lose weight, and what changes within you with the passing of time, you will be able to transform inspiration into motivation. Transformation is the willingness to be open to change. And, the challenge to motivation is to be able to sustain this process.

As the source of your motivation is derived from something you were inspired to do, lets go back and examine some of the qualities of inspiration. Inspiration is that exhilarating state that makes you feel that anything is possible. It is a state that accesses powerful images and feelings. These images and feelings are the result of identifying all the qualities and benefits that losing weight will bring you.

The primary reason why inspiration is so ephemeral is that it is difficult to sustain such passionate feelings and acute impressions. If we step down the energy of level of 'inspiration' a number of notches, we get 'motivation'.

In order to be able to lose weight you need to be able to turn *inspiration* into *motivation*. You need to be able to recall and *re-create the source to your inspiration* on a continuing basis.

As you move through your daily life you draw on different sources for motivation. One form of incentive is that of being motivated by some source outside of yourself. This may a photograph in a magazine, or a personal compliment from a friend.

Another form of motivation is a response to your inner needs. This form of motivation is of a deeper nature and concerns being able to meaningfully find expression to your life. Both forms of motivation are necessary to losing weight, both serve you in different ways.

The first of these, is referred to as External Motivation.

External Motivation

External motivation concerns motivational images that are derived from sources outside of yourself. When you see someone with a beautiful body, or see a photograph of yourself before you put on weight and this stimulates you to want change, then this is what is referred to as external motivation. External motivation is an effective means of helping you to achieve your goals. One of the many ways that you can use this form of motivation is to cut out pictures that inspire you. You may cut out different body parts of people that you admire. It is often a good idea not to show the persons face. Compose your picture so that it stimulates you to want change. These pictures can then be stuck to your cupboard door, or any other prominent spot in your home.

Like all forms of stimuli it is important to become aware of the responses that these stimuli elicit - for it is not so much the picture that inspires you, but the **thought of the qualities and benefits that these things will bring you.** The more you associate these benefits with your need to lose weight, the more motivated you will be to achieve.

The other form of motivation that is essential to achieving your vision of a slim and healthy body is Internal Motivation.

Internal Motivation

Whereas external motivation deals with externally derived inspirational images, internal motivation is a state of inner energy that emanates from your core needs, your deeper desires. This energy helps keep you focused and directed towards attaining your visions.

To discover what these core needs are, you need to ask the question: What is the essence to my need? Do you want to lose weight because it will make you happy, or is it because you think it will improve your health? For example, you may think that losing weight will make you happier. You may discover that in fact you can achieve the happiness you desire through improving your relationship with your partner, or by changing your career path. It is important to uncover your true motives for wanting to lose weight, and if in fact there are alternative ways for achieving this intention.

On getting clear on your intention, the following questions must be asked: What is losing weight going to do for me? In what way will it make me feel different? How will it improve my life?

It is important to get clear on what it is that you want from losing weight. Do you want beauty, health, love, admiration? Define the qualities of what you want. Is there some other way that you can achieve these things? Being crystal clear on your *core* reasons will assist you in being motivated to lose weight.

Spend as much time as you need. Write down your motives for wanting to lose weight.

....

....

....

....

Is there any other way that you could obtain these qualities without having to lose weight? Could you find security, happiness, confidence etc., by improving your beliefs, or through your job or relationship/s? It is vital that you discover exactly what your underlying needs are.

....
....
....
....

Summarize what you have learnt about motivation:

....
....
....
....

Being motivated to lose weight requires that you have an effective strategy - an inspired vision of what you want to attain.

Vision Setting

By the age of 37 he was regarded as one of the wealthiest men in America. The corporation he co-founded employs some 12,000 employees and generates billions of dollars in sales every year.[2] If you have not already guessed, the man is none other than Bill Gates the president of Microsoft Corporation, the largest supplier of computer operating soft-

---

[2] From an article entitled "Just an ordinary guy" in Excellence Magazine Spring 1992

ware systems for personal computers in the world. All of this began with a vision, an inspired vision of the future.

In 1975 - six years before the first IBM personal computer hit the market - Gates and Microsoft co-founder Paul Allen wrote out a vision to inspire themselves: 'A personal computer on every desk and in every home'.

Would Bill Gates have achieved all this without a vision? Would he have been able to pursue his dream so single-mindedly and brilliantly without a vision of the future? It was this vision of *'A personal computer on every desk and in every home'* that enabled Bill Gates to build a software empire.

Setting visions assists you in defining exactly what you want from life. Visions focus your intentions and enable you to create a clear picture of what you want in the future. Vision is the 'act of seeing'. In this context, the act, or faculty of seeing, relates to how you view yourself in the future and more importantly, what this will do for you. For it is not simply a matter of losing weight and creating a beautiful body, but what qualities and benefits you will receive as a result of losing weight.

Setting visions not only gives you something to aim at, it implants a strong directive to your subconscious mind. This directive continues to send 'thin' messages to your body long after you have forgotten about your vision of being slim.

Over the years I have on numerous occasions toyed with this amazing phenomena of the mind - the power of suggestion. The basis to my experimentation was to set a vision to lose a specific amount of weight over a given period of time. I would for example determine that I wanted to lose six and a half pounds (3 Kg.) over a period of say three months. The procedure I then followed was to be crystal clear about my intention. I was totally unequivocal about what I wanted and my reasons for wanting to lose weight. I would then focus on my vision repeatedly for a period of one to two weeks. After this period I made no conscious effort to continue focusing on my vision. If by chance it happened to come up for me, well and good. If not, it didn't matter. Another important condition to this exercise was that I made no effort to alter my approach to eating. I made no attempt to diet down, or increase my exercise. My approach was to continue normally with my life. At the end of the period I then weighed myself. On all the occasions that I attempted to lose weight by setting a defined vision - a clear intention, the results were always approximately within thirty percent of my target weight. On some occasions it was dead on target. (It must be noted that my target weight was always a realistically set goal). The suggestive potential of vision setting clearly indicates the potential and power of the mind.

Vision setting assists you in attaining what you want from life. The key to vision setting is to establish exactly what you want.

Before you can even begin to consider losing weight and creating your ideal body, it is essential to establish a clear vision of what you really want. The clearer your vision the quicker you will actualize weight loss. Vision setting can be defined as those visions that are general and those that are specific.

A general vision would be; "I want to lose weight", or "I would love to have a beautiful figure". On the other hand a specific vision would be; "I want to lose 8 pounds (3.6 Kg.) by the end of September", or, " I want to lose three inches around my hips". Being specific sharpens your visions. This acuity gives you the power and intention to attain the results you want.

Lets begin by starting to put together your vision. To create your ideal figure, how much weight would you need to lose?

....

How long do you realistically expect it to take you to lose this weight?

....

What do you expect losing this weight will do for you? Will it give you beauty, health, self-love, admiration, self-confidence?

....

....

....

Are there any other ways you can achieve these qualities, without having to lose weight?

....

....

....

....

How passionately do you want to lose weight?

....

What would you have to do to improve your lifestyle?

....

....

....

....

Dreams and creative imagination can greatly contribute to attaining your visions. For example, you may have a dream of your perfect body. Any form of creative imagination stimulates and assists in defining your vision. The more specific your images are, the more focused your vision.

Your Body Vision

Let's zone in now and specify your 'body vision'. Working through each body part, determine how important it is for you to improve each part, and how this relates to your vision of what you want to achieve.

(Use a rating system of 1 - 3; 1 being very important and 3 being not so important).

Body Part	Rating	Specific Vision

Vision setting should be a fun process. Vision setting is an effortless process - it differs from goal setting in that there is no implicit pressure for you to have to succeed. And, as such no anticipated feelings of failure. Visions merely set direction to your intention/s; they help to channel your creative energy.

You may find that sometimes you experience an energy block when setting visions. You may find that conflicting emotions come up for you. You may emotionally experience this as depression, or confusion. If this should happen there is no need to try and deny these feelings. Simply observe your feelings without trying to suppress them. Feel into the problem and see if you can sense what it is you are not seeing. You will usually discover that if you move beyond the issue and rather focus on the energy behind the problem, you will begin to see the solution. As Jack Schwartz in his book *Voluntary Controls* so wisely states: *"Every time a problem is born, its solution is created too."* This awareness will dissipate the negative energy. Once these feelings have subsided, continue with putting down what you want to attain.

As you practice vision setting you will experience the joy of creating.

Summarize your short term vision (1day - 1 month) of how you wish your body to look: choose those visions that you feel you can realistically and comfortably attain. Quite often we seek visions that we really have no intention of attaining. We are more attached to the process of pursuing our visions than actually achieving them. The question must be asked; "Am I prepared to accept this completely?"

Short term visions give you a sense of your ability to begin losing weight. By attempting to first lose small amounts of weight you are then encouraged to expand your future visions.

Short-Term Visions

Set down your vision for tomorrow.

....

....

....

Establish your vision for next week.

....

....

....

....

Now plan your vision for the next three weeks.

....

....

....

....

Having defined your visions, what are you going to do to attain these visions? What specific actions are you going to take?

....

....

....

....

Medium-Term Visions

Now having done this summarize your medium term vision (1 - 6 months): Take your short term visions and magnify them. Sense your potential to attain and expand your visions. Summarizing your medium term vision assists you in defining your longer term visions.

....

....

....

....

Long-term Visions

Stretch your imagination even further. Create your long-term vision of how you wish to look (6 months - 48 months). By creating these long term visions you are recognizing that visions have the ability to manifest if you desire them to. Even though you may be giving free reign to your imagination, your long term vision should relate to what you want from your short term vision.

....

....

....

....

....

Do not worry about what you have written down. Visions are flexible, you can always come back some time in the future and re-adjust your visions.
    Vision setting includes the recognition that beyond our personal aspirations lies an intention that is far deeper and more vital than what meets the eye. This recognition enfolds the understanding that everything happens for a purpose. All you need

to do is to see the 'connection'. There will be times when you wish to achieve something and no matter what you do you are unable to make the situation work. These are the times that you need to acknowledge that you are being guided on a course that may not appear to align with your intended vision. In these instances you need to recognize that above your mental, emotional, and physical intentions, rests your spiritual intention. It is this 'purpose' that calls to be integrated into your visions. For, everything that 'happens' to us is leading us forward in our quest for attainment. It may appear to fly in the face of what we may have intended, but the mere fact that these so called 'negative' situations generally persist is indication of their significance. If we can but just learn to appreciate, to accept this aspect of our personal advancement we can make the attunement necessary for the attainment of harmony and fulfilment.

Visions merely provide a guideline for attainment. The other important point to remember is that you must only put down what you *really* want, not what you wishfully think you want.

How do you know when you have energized your vision sufficiently? When you envisage something and you can almost feel it coming then you are exercising the desirable amount of energy. On the other hand, if what you want seems distant and more like a wish than an actuality then you are employing too little energy. It is not necessary to over-expend energy on vision setting, or anything else for that matter. All that is required is the necessary input - no less, no more. Begin initially with setting visions that are relevant and attainable.

As you become more attuned you will be able to expand your visions to all areas of your life. Establishing visions means that within your order of needs there will be some visions that are more important than others. This necessitates that you are able to prioritise your visions so that they are relevant and attainable.

Prioritising

During the day you are faced with numerous choices as to how best expend your time and energy. You are faced with the demands of your career, how you spend your leisure time, and many other considerations that make up the full spectrum of daily experience. At another level you also have dreams and visions. How you allocate your personal resources determines how effectively and timeously you achieve these visions. The key to achieving is being able to prioritise; the ability to effectively allocate your time and energy.

If you were a jogger and you wished to run a 26 mile (42 Km.) marathon you would need to prioritise. Your daily training would necessitate that you run an average of 5 - 6 miles (8 - 10 Km.) per day. On the weekend you would need to run a total of approximately 25 miles (40 Km.). For a period of at least 4 - 6 months prior to running your race you would have to dedicate yourself to training. This may entail curtailing your social activities so that you could get up early in the morning to train. You would need to eat correctly and strategize your training. The numerous demands for achieving your vision would require that you would have to put some of your other visions and needs on hold.

One of the most effective ways to achieve a vision is to prioritise. *Prioritising focuses your resources on what you want to achieve most.* It does not mean that you need to abandon your other visions permanently, it simply means that for the necessary period of time you need to be completely centred on your primary vision; in this case your primary vision is to lose weight and create your body beautiful and vital.

Losing weight requires that for an initial period you need to devote as much of your energy and personal resources to attaining your intended vision. This means making a commitment - a commitment to positively affirming your ability to lose weight, directing your thoughts and emotions, and being sensitive to your bodies nutritional needs. Prioritising does not necessitate 'efforting'. It really means being focused so that you are not distracted by other needs. It means acknowledging the fact that you have choices, and that the choice you make concerns losing weight.

To get clear on your priorities jot down your answers to the following questions:

What is the purpose of prioritising?

....

....

....

List your three most important priorities.

....

....

....

Now list these in order of priority.

1: ....

2: ....

3: ....

Ask yourself the following question: Are you prepared to focus all your energies on your number one priority until you achieve your vision?

(YES/NO) ....

Do you also appreciate that at a later stage you will be able to return to your other visions?

(YES/NO) ....

If weight-loss is your number one priority, how much time and energy will you need to devote to achieving your vision of weight-loss?

....

....

....

It is simply not enough to make a decision to lose weight. To be propelled into action you need to be *moved* to want to make new choices. You need to be passionate about wanting to lose weight.

Passion Power

I am sure if I asked you to think of something that you really love you would respond with passion. Passion is that deep 'love of'; it is a powerful emotion that fires you to be deeply stimulated to take action. It is that soaring feeling that elevates your thoughts, that drives you to want to attain. Mozart had passion, Einstein, Gauguin, and Nureyev had passion - *you have passion!* In fact anyone who is out there attaining in some meaningful way has passion.

Passion is that feeling that gives birth to all that is great. Passion is the one quality we all have in abundance - it is what enables us to ignite our dreams with energy.

Passion is the aspiration to fly, rather than crawl, to be slim and healthy rather than overweight. Passion means loving yourself and your body so much that you are willing to examine your eating patterns and thought processes. It is the need to direct your life rather than aimlessly meander from situation to situation.

So much for passion, but how does one create passion? Passion is something that once you locate you can return to as often as you like. The source of passion is love: a love that emanates from a deep and abiding recognition of that which is wonderful. Passion is an overpowering affection of the mind, and of the heart. When you truly love someone or something, you are passionate. And, in this, you are magnanimous and expansive in your thoughts, feelings and actions. It is these qualities that precipitate greatness.

When you begin to recognize and acknowledge who, and what you are, you trigger your potential to be passionate. As you explore your potential and discover your empowerment, your passion for attainment will increase exponentially.

What do you truly love in your life?

....

....

....

What is it about this that you love? What are the qualities that being passionate brings to you?

....

....

....

How does this feel? What feelings do you associate with this passion?

....

....

....

Try and locate where you feel this passion.

....

How do you feel passion can motivate you to achieve your vision of losing weight ?

....

....

....

....

If you are passionate about wanting to lose weight then this will be your foremost commitment. This commitment will enable you to direct your resources, one of which is - the Essence of Time.

The Essence of Time

It is only by time that we are separated from our desires.   Herman Hesse

Time is the essence to change and there is no time like the moment to begin.
    When we consider change we always look to the future and determine to do something one day. All that happens is that time passes, time that could have been used to begin the process that would have brought you to where you are now.
    'Personal' time has a strange psychological warp to it. If you look forward in time when you are

considering taking action, it seems interminable. If from the same point you look back in time it seems to be foreshortened. Similarly, depending on your mood time appears slower or faster. If you are enjoying what you are doing time appears to go faster. On the other hand if you dislike what you are doing time seems to drag. Thus, when you consider initiating change you may be confronted by the feeling, "I've got so much weight to lose and it is going to take me so long that I do not know that I feel like going through all of this". What in effect you have done is to mentally create a picture of *stretched* future time. Attached to this is a string of negative emotional associations. Even though it is possibly only going to take you three or four months to lose the weight, the fact that you are dealing with future time means that the idea of losing weight becomes psychologically burdensome. So when we speak of time we are implying that time is 3-dimensional i.e. that time has duration, direction and velocity.

Stop thinking that one day you will suddenly feel motivated to lose weight. The timeless excuse that all you really need to do is to resolve your current problems and then you will be ready to do something about your life, is another of the many distractions you create in evading what needs doing now. Fear of failure is yet another illusion of the mind. You can go on creating reasons interminably.

"Whether its the best of times or the worst of times, its the only time you've got".   Art Buchwald

The essence to facing time is be in the moment. Make your decision to initiate movement by focusing on your available personal resources rather than on future time and its limiting emotional responses. When you are faced with giving a time value to something that you wish to achieve, like how long it is going to take you to lose the required weight, picture time as being vertical rather than horizontal. Visualize the moment as moving effortlessly upwards in time rather than a point that is moving interminably out towards the horizon. Future and past time in reality do not exist, they only exist as concepts of the mind. Attainment too is a vertical process. It is more an ascendancy than a movement along the plane of horizontality.

Time, like all resources demands that you do not squander your opportunities. The old time worn adage aptly sums up delaying what needs doing now, *Procrastination is the thief of time.* We all only have 24 hours in our day. You never hear those that are achieving complaining that they do not have enough time to their day!

Invest your time now and earn interest for the future. The sooner you begin acting out your visions, the sooner you will enjoy the benefits. *Taking action becomes a self-fulfilling process.* If you fail to act now time merely acts to repeat the same old patterns.

Another aspect of time that limits our ability to attain is that we have a notion that 'everything takes time'. There is no natural law that states that the passage of time is essential to personal change. Only you decide how much time it is going to take to lose weight.

Personal transformation takes as little, or as much time as you deem necessary. The constraint of time is imposed from within, not from without. If you are prepared to face the issue of losing weight and involve your whole being in the process of personal transformation you can instantaneously begin enacting change.

The Ebb and Flow Cycle

Life is not made up of one uninterrupted movement. Movement is created through the rhythm of ebb and flow - through cycles of growth and rest.

These cycles or rhythms, are the basic pattern to all of life. Periods of stimulatory growth are always followed by periods of energy shifts that appear to be of a somewhat dormant nature. In effect what is really happening is that this is the ebb part of the ebb and flow cycle. This is the downbeat to the cadence of energy. It is the preparatory stage that is necessary for the next spurt of personal growth and change.

The process of the ebb and flow is a continuum that is made up of differing rhythms. In nature the cycles of hot and cold, day and night, summer and winter are analogous to our own cycles of personal growth. At a biological level our bodies resonate to these rhythms in what we refer to as our biorhythms and circadian rhythms. The principle of ebb and flow is also marvellously mirrored in the human nervous system which is attuned to the steady variance of action and rest.

Going with the flow as the saying goes, enables you to channel your energy effectively. Resistance to either part of the cycle merely impedes your ability to achieve.

One of the central underlying characteristics of ancient Tao philosophy is that all growth in nature is determined by the cyclical patterns of coming and going. The Taoist symbols of yin and yang characterize the dynamic cyclical aspect that constitutes all physical and human growth.

"The yang having reached its climax retreats in favour of the yin; the yin having reached it climax retreats in favour of the yang."[3]

It appears that cycles underlie all aspects of nature. Even at an atomic level energy is punctuated. Max Planck, the founding father of the quantum theory, discovered that in fact atoms radiate energy in spurts. Atoms appear to emit and absorb energy in determinate amounts. What Planck was able to establish was that *"the changes of nature are 'explosive', not continuous and smooth"*.[4]

So the next time you experience a 'down' to what you have charted as your course, whether it be losing weight or achieving at work or any other area of your life, get a sense of the different types of energy that are at work in your life. Realize that the dormant phases are preparing you for the next stage of growth and that each phase is determined by the preceding one. Being attuned to the pulse of your life ensures that you will achieve what you set out to do.

Re-framing

One of the most powerful approaches to effective personal change is the notion of re-framing - the ability to change your frame of reference and in so doing change the meaning. If you can change the meaning,

---

[3] Wang Ch'ung quoted in *Science and Civilization in China* by J.Needham published by Cambridge University Press.
[4] *The Dancing Wu Li Masters* by Gary Zukav published by Rider.

you change your response. And, if you can change your response, you change the result.

Re-framing is inextricably linked to personal creativity. Like all creative processes, re-framing is about being able to come from a different position, a position of openness and expansiveness.

Re-framing is not a new idea. The alchemists of old talked of turning dross into gold, a re-frame that embodies spiritual change. You often hear the expression, "It all depends on how you frame the situation." How you frame something determines the meaning you attach to it.

The basic notion of *Fat Equals Thin* is in fact a re-frame. *Fat Equals Thin* embraces the concept of being able to creatively view the behavioral patterns that created you overweight, in a new and enabling way. This re-frame empowers you to transform *Fat* into *Thin*.

Re-framing literally means placing a larger more expansive frame around an issue; being able to enlarge and change your frame of reference and in so doing, change your response. If you take your problem and place it in a small frame it becomes all-consuming. Take this same problem and place a large frame around it that includes all the other aspects that make up the full spectrum of your life and you diminish the size of your problem. Your problem simply becomes one of the many parts that make up your personal landscape.

All issues, all situations carry the potential for being viewed from different vantage points. They can be viewed as an opportunity for personal growth or personal defeat. You can frame any situation either positively or negatively. Adversity can represent either a gift or a handicap, it all depends on what it means to you!

I am sure if you think back on your life you will recall situations that appeared at first to be an insurmountable problem, but by being able to look at the situation from a different viewpoint, by being able to re-frame, you were able to turn this around. What springs readily to mind are those situations where one is involved in a personal confrontation with either a friend, partner or work colleague. Generally ones first response is to self-justify - they are wrong, and you are right. Once your emotions have settled you are able to place a different frame around the situation. By being more expansive you are able to see other dimensions to the situation. You are able to see that the situation is not merely a personal affront, but rather about being able to include the other person's viewpoint. By placing a larger frame around the situation you are able to see added dimensions that change what the situation means to you. The result of this is that you are able to respond differently. You have choices which now empower rather than limit you.

Re-framing embodies being able to understand how to effectively replace a behaviour that you find limiting with a behaviour that is more enabling. Re-framing encompasses the recognition that every part of you serves a function. Beyond the concept of polar opposites like 'good' or 'bad', 'right' or 'wrong', 'this' or 'that', resides the recognition that everything is part of a whole and as such serves a purpose. Even anger in certain situations serves a function. Given a life-threatening situation anger can assist in warding off a would be aggressor. If one of your many *parts* has the need to overeat this does not necessarily mean it is bad. Yes, certainly it leads to a condition of overweight, but reframed the intention of this pattern could serve you well. By changing the frame you change the pattern.

Re-framing acknowledges that it is necessary to honour whatever behavioral pattern you display. In some intrinsic way all behaviour serves you. What is important is to recognize that there may be other alternative behavioral responses that may serve you better. Re-framing is about choice, it is about being able to expand your behavioral responses. Once you are able to understand what the underlying intention is that propels you to overeat (in other words what this part is doing for you) you have the choice of fulfilling this intention in some other meaningful way. But, until you are able to understand what this part is doing for you, you cannot simply discard it. Re-framing is not about discarding any behavioral pattern, rather it concerns being able to find other more acceptable forms of behaviour that fulfil the same intention.

Re-framing at one level means being able to see a broader perspective - being able to view a situation dimensionally. At another, it encompasses the means to replace a behavioral pattern with other choices that you find more acceptable. Behavioral patterns like binging or overeating are linked to an inner need, whether this be fear, anxiety, dissatisfaction, disillusionment or any other emotion. The process of re-framing enables you to create alternative behaviours that are more effective at fulfilling these needs.

Personal Potential

Since his early twenties he has had to live with amyotrophic lateral sclerosis, a slow degenerative disease that results in the disintegration of the nerve cells in the spinal cord and brain. His list of personal and scientific achievements are sufficient to convince anyone of his brilliance and courage. He is unable to walk, feed himself or perform any other normal function. At the age of thirty-eight he was inaugurated as the Lucasian Professor of Mathematics, a position once held by Sir Isaac Newton. His Theory of Everything and work done on the Black Holes are but a few of the scientific breakthroughs that he is associated with.

Regarded as one of the most brilliant and expansive theoretical physicists since Einstein, Stephen Hawking was able to potentialize his predicament. Granted, Stephen was born with the gift of a brilliant and incisive mind, but given his enormous physical disability he could quite easily have given in to depression and despair. In fact there were many periods when his physical disability did get to him but Stephen always managed to turn this around. Whether it be raising a family or coping with the enormous difficulty of merely trying to express himself Stephen Hawking's story is one of acknowledging what he had rather than what he did not have.

Potential is another of your unlimited resources. It is only limited by your belief systems.

As unique individuals we are all endowed differently. For example, one person may have a faster metabolism, another may have an aptitude for mathematics. Each of us is unique in this aspect. If we take what we have and develop this there is so much we can achieve. No one has ever exhausted their potential. What you are endowed with can be transformed and developed endlessly.

Potential refers to any area of your life and includes some of the following aspects:
- the potential to lose weight and improve your body shape
- the potential to be filled with health and vitality
- the potential to love and appreciate yourself and others unconditionally
- the potential to be great at your job
- the potential to be considerate and giving
- the potential to direct your life
- the potential to find happiness and joy
- the potential to find spiritual fulfilment

Add to the above list all those aspects of your potentiality that you feel will assist you to lose weight and direct your life:

....

....

....

....

Is there any impediment that prevents you from realizing your potential, other than the way in which you view yourself?

....

You can potentialize any situation. Often individuals realize their potential under pressure or through adversity. Stephen Hawking is but one example of this. One of the great opportunities that enables you to realize your potential is that of being overweight.

Being overweight is a wonderful opportunity for examining and developing those potentials and abilities you may have never considered. It is an opportunity to recognize your potentiality. Facing your condition gives you the opportunity for developing self-awareness, resourcefulness, and self-love.

Losing weight is only part of something much bigger - it is the catalyst that creates the exchange of growth. Losing weight not only offers you the benefits of beauty, health and vitality, it also serves a higher purpose. It is a time in which you merge with your soul. It is a time in which you reach inward and upward. That is why you need to recognize that you did not just become fat. You created this condition for the elevated purpose of expanded growth.

Being able to view matters from an elevated viewpoint gives you a far bigger perspective than if you view the issue from the ground. The more expansive your vista, the greater the potential for personal growth. Even though the primary intention of this book is to assist you in losing weight, facing overweight is an opportunity to open up other cardinal areas of your life. It is an opportunity to realize your unlimited potential.

Potential is developed when you are prepared to stretch yourself beyond that which you normally believe possible. This includes being open to new ideas and approaches.

By involving yourself in the process of losing weight you are tapping your potential. If you choose you can lose whatever weight is necessary to create your body the way you want it. This unbounded aspect is one of your most dynamic and exciting attributes. Potential is a gift that obliges you to benefit from its promise.

Chapter Seven

Eating for Pleasure

Dieting can be represented by the three big D's - **Deprivation, Discipline and Desire.** Dieting sets up a sequence of chain-reactions that eventually leads to frustration and finally, failure.

As a concept dieting implies that you deprive yourself of certain foods, or quantities thereof in order to lose weight. This requires that you be disciplined in your eating habits. Discipline in turn demands enforcement. Enforcement necessitates suppression. Any form of suppression must inevitably create inner conflict....and inner conflict leads to preoccupation, fixation, or obsession with that which you are denying. Can you remember the last time that you denied yourself something you wanted? What happened? I bet that all that you could think of was that which you were denying! Eventually you must rebel and break your diet. This is followed by guilt..... and guilt by yet more inner turmoil.

The more you attempt to deny what you feel the more you energize that inclination. The fact that there is a battle between your desires and your resolve to be disciplined, means that as soon as something in your life does not work out you are going to look for an excuse to go back to your old eating patterns.

So what you have done, is that through attempting to diet you have set yourself up to fail. Actually it is not **you** that fails, rather it is **dieting** that fails!

Even if you are successful at initially losing weight there is still the consideration of being able to sustain this weight loss. Statistics reveal that 98% of all dieters regain all the weight they lost, plus interest.[1] In fact, science now tells us that losing and gaining weight repeatedly increases one of the enzymes (lipoprotein lipase) that advances storage of fat. So, at all levels dieting leads to failure.

Diets are prescriptive. In some way or another they prescribe 'what', or 'how much' you should eat, or both. As unique and differing individuals our needs vary. My needs are not your needs.

This brings us to a fundamental consideration, there is no single 'universal' dietary approach that works for everyone. What produces results for you may not produce results for another. What you require is a nutritional approach that works for *'you'*. This approach must fit your lifestyle, personality, biochemical and physiological needs. Inasmuch as there is no single approach to losing weight that works for everyone, so there are no specific foods that work all of the time. What may prove effective for one period, may not continue to produce the results for another. You need a dynamic approach that changes from day to day, week to week, and month to month.

Living embodies movement, and as such involves continual change. Not only are you influenced by your body's bio-rhythms but as you go about your day what you mentally, emotionally, physically and spiritually experience determines what you need to

---

[1] *Overcoming Overeating* by Jane R. Hirschmann and Carol Munter, published by Cedar.

eat. Sitting on the beach is not quite the same experience as facing a business or personal crisis!

The basis to our thinking in the West is deeply aligned with science. This rub-off has in part contributed to the way in which we view our bodies. The notion that we are essentially made up of immutable matter rather than dynamic resonating fields of energy, has influenced not only the way in which we look at ourselves, but also our notion of what we should eat.

This 'mechanistic' perception carries with it the attendant inference that the body be regarded as a biochemical and physiological constant. Our assumption of diet is based on a corresponding concept. And this is where we arrive at a very important point; the basis to all diets is that they are formulated by certain fixed principles. Thus by implication, any form of dieting or fixed conceptual approach must entail a certain degree of rigidity. Rigidity denies the dynamics of individuality.

The only way to align with your rhythms and varying needs is to eat what you need - **to eat intuitively.** Through being in tune with your four bodies you have the ability to *'intuitively'* pick up on the continuous play of information being relayed to you by your holistic body. For encoded within your being is the intelligence necessary for a profound knowing of what is needed from moment to moment.

Where nutritional science leaves off your innate intuition and intelligence takes off. Through developing your higher intelligence (intuition), you will discover that you are both scientist and laboratory in your own physical and metaphysical world. What you discover will prove to you that you have the means to promote health and sustain lasting weight loss.

> ### The Diet Loop!
> Dieting requires that you be disciplined, that you do not eat certain foods. This suppression creates inner conflict which leads to preoccupation with that which you are denying. Denial inevitably leads you to break out and go back to your old eating patterns.

'You' - the Dynamic Individual

Medical science has made great strides in reducing nutrition to broad principles. These principles constitute a vast body of knowledge, but when interfaced with the constantly changing dynamics of the individual condition the limitations of these principles soon becomes apparent. Nutrition is not only a complex and intricate affair, it is often an indeterminate and inexact business. Not only are there differing *expert* opinions on the subject but there are also vast areas that still form part of the unknown. This state of affairs is further compounded by factors such as; synergy, hereditary factors, current health status, environment, exercise, bioavailabilty of nutrients, excretion of nutrition, to mention but a few. All influence and affect your nutritional status.

"The reason that there is no single caloric formula for weight loss (or weight gain, for that matter) is that individual metabolisms differ. What is optimal

for one person concerning food intake may simply be inadequate for another."[2]

Nutrition is a complex set of varying factors. Medical science considers between 40 and 60 nutrients (depending on the authority's terms of reference) to constitute the range of what is essential for the sustenance of life. These nutrients are generally comprised of 8 - 11 amino acids, 2 essential fatty acids, 13 vitamins, 22 minerals, water, fibre, and energy that is derived from fats and carbohydrates.

Nutrients are thus regarded as either essential or non-essential. If the body is incapable of manufacturing the nutrient it is regarded as essential. Even in this area medical science is continually re-appraising what constitutes an essential nutrient. For a long time vitamin E and the mineral zinc were not regarded as essential nutrients. Today their vital importance is recognized. There are many other examples of scientific re-assessment. Dr Michael Colgan, one of the leading experts in nutritional science includes in his latest assessment of vital nutrients, 6 co-factors or helper substances. In another essential area he reveals *"The fact that your body can get by on 10 amino acids and can manufacture the rest does not mean that it will do so effectively. Generating the other 10 amino acids required to build muscle, for instance, demands a lot of your biochemistry."[3]* Dr. Colgan goes on to quote medical studies done on patients with degenerative muscle disorders. These studies reveal that patients fed doses of essential amino ac-

---

[2] From an article by Ronald S.Laura PhD. and Kenneth R.Dutton PhD *Protein Loading -Muscle and Fitness* June 1992
[3] From an article by Michael Colgan PhD entitled *Amino Acids* in the June 1995 edition of Muscle and Fitness

ids in correct proportion but not including a balance of non-essential aminos, excreted most of the supplemented essential amino's. Instead of improving the patients continued to lose muscle. So, maybe our evaluation of essential amino acids needs to be extended to include 20 or even 22 amino acids!

Like all definitions, the summation of what constitutes an essential nutrient is based on what is necessary for maintaining a state of existence. Once again the rigidity of this definition falls short of including optimum health. As in the case of amino acids, a more expanded approach to nutrition is needed. The needs and demands of a rapidly changing world within which we all live necessitates that our view be as inclusive and broad as possible.

Having briefly touched on what medical science defines as essential nutrients, it is now necessary to extend our line of questioning. Answers to some of the following questions need to be given: What constitutes an optimum rather than just an adequate state of health? Nutritionally what is needed to achieve this? The answers to this set of complex questions are determined in part by the guidelines established by the country's national Food and Nutrition Board. These guidelines are generally referred to as the Recommended Dietary/Daily Allowance, or RDA.

The RDA Factor

RDA's are intended to form the basis of what is nutritionally necessary for adequate health and general well-being. It is also interesting to note that RDA'S are based on the needs of sedentary individuals, and make no allowance for factors such as, illness and exercise. It must also be noted that the line of argument that is being developed here essentially demands that *adequate* be replaced by *optimum* for we are concerned with soaring rather than crawling. The sample of RDA's below illustrate the assessments of different countries.

Recommended dietary intakes for adults.

	Aus	Ca	Ger	Ne	Sw	UK	USA	Rus
female							800	
Vit. A	750		900	450	900	750		1500
(ug) male		999					999	
female					55			64
Vit.C	30	30	75	50		30	45	
(mg) male					60			75
female		1.4	1.8	0.8	1.0	0.9	1.0	1.5
Thiamine	1.1							
(mg) male		1.0	1.4	1.0	1.4	1.1	1.4	1.8
female	700	800	700					
Calcium				800	800	500	800	800
(mg) male	800	800	800					
female	15	14	18	12	18	12	18	
Iron								15
(mg) male	12	10	12	10	10	10	10	

Key: Au Australia; **Ca** Canada; **Ger** Germany; **Ne** Netherlands; **Sw** Sweden; **UK** United Kingdom; **USA** United States of America; **Rus** Russia.
Source for Table: *Thorson's Complete Guide to Vitamins and minerals* by Leonard Mervyn

If we now compare the above figures it is quite clear that in some instances there is a fairly large discrepancy between some of the countries. A number of questions arise out of these obvious differentials. The first of these is: if these levels are established through scientific assessment - why the discrepancy? The obvious answer to this must be simply that nutrition is not an exact science. What one body or authority evaluates as being nutritionally sufficient does not necessarily correlate with another.

The second question concerns what constitutes a 'healthy person'. The American Food and Nutrition Board defines this as: *"A state of complete physical, mental and social well-being and not merely the absence of disease or infirmity."*

If the RDA's of nutrients are sufficient for the promotion of complete health - why are there so few well people? I am sure you will be hard pressed to think of someone who is not prone to sore throats, headaches, colds, sore ears, or many of the other common ailments that so afflict us. Optimum health includes not only being free of any ailment, but embodies also being possessed of vitality and sound mind.

Thirdly, what do these RDA's mean to you and I? If RDA's are incapable of assuring a state of complete health and well-being what is their value? The recognition that the RDA's of vitamins, minerals, amino acids and energy giving nutrients are necessary for existence cannot be denied. But these levels of nutritional intake in themselves do not assure a state of optimum health that we all so desire. We must therefore draw the conclusion that RDA's be regarded as a general guideline to the issue of nutrition.

One of the many other dynamic facets of nutrition that requires consideration is that of synergy - the absorbtion, assimilation and utilization of nutrients. Synergy suggests that every nutrient has the capacity to affect the action of all other nutrients. In other words, nutrients do not interact in a singular and simple way, but rather *"... interlock in an incredibly complex set of inter-relating pathways, varying with time and with different parts of the body. Each essential nutrient interlocks, either directly or indirectly, with every other nutrient."*[4] For example:

- Vitamin D which assists in promoting the absorbtion of calcium.
- Magnesium which plays a part in the metabolism of vitamin C, phosphorous, sodium and potassium.
- The family of B vitamins which are far more potent when synergistically combined than when used separately.
- Vitamin E deficiency increases deficiency in zinc, which in turn increase the body's levels of copper.

This scenario is further complicated by the fact that your individual biochemical needs too are unique. For not only are the molecular functions of individual cells different, but even your glands, organs and muscles differ in size to that of another. Extensive research by Professor R. Williams at the University of Texas illustrates quite clearly the widely divergent nutritional needs of individuals. For example, the bodily usage of vitamin A can vary as much as 40-

---

[4] *What's in my Food* by Xandria Williams published by Prism Press.

fold.[5] The issue of nutrition is further complicated by illness and stress.

No matter how we view nutrition, we are inevitably channelled back to the undeniable recognition that each person is not only dynamic, but also unique. This being so, how do diets fit into the scheme of things?

The Diet!

Diets are formulated either generally or specifically. Those that are more general, offer you a set of principals which if adhered to promise weight loss and in some cases even the added bonus of energy and wellbeing. Those that are more specific calculate the calorie intake required to reach a specified target weight. Both approaches, whether they be general or specific are dependant on the adherence to a set of fixed principles.

Any approach that in some way or another prescribes what, or how you must eat, must at some point break down. (The author acknowledges that obviously different diets employ different principles and approaches.) The point that needs making, is that any *definitive* concept that does not take into account the diverse and varying needs of the individual cannot fulfil the essential criteria of:

- **effortless weight loss**
- **sustainable weight loss**
- **optimum health.**

---

[5] *Optimum Sports Nutrition: Your Competitive Edge - A Complete Guide for Optimizing Athletic Performance* by Dr.Michael Colgan published by Colgan - Amino Research

The underlying principal to all forms of weight loss is the apparently simple equation of what you eat versus what you burn off, whether the method of losing weight be the F-Plan Diet (fibre based diet), High Protein Diet, Stillman Diet, Scarsdale Diet, Carbohydrate Cravers, Beverly Hills Diet, or any one of the numerous other dietary approaches. If you consume more than your body can burn off you will get fat!

In order to be able to calculate what your daily caloric consumption should be to enable you to lose weight it is first necessary to assess how much weight you need to lose. This is determined by establishing your ideal or target weight. There are a number of ways that this is done. One of the methods is that your ideal weight is arrived at from comparing your height, age and gender to a chart of established body weights.

Alternatively, your relative leanness is derived from measuring your weight against your height giving you your Body Mass Index, or BMI. From this the Body Fat Percentage (BFP) is calculated. More accurate methods of determining your BFP, include Underwater Weighing, the Dual Photon Absorptiometry test, Bioelectrical Impedence Analysis, Total Body Electrical Conductivity and the Skin-Fold Callipers. Even though these various forms of testing enable you to measure how much fat your body contains in relation to muscle and lean body mass, the *"body composition experts agree that no single test is perfect"*[6]

---

[6] From an article *Fat Guage* in Allure January 199..by Lucy Danziger.

Once you have determined how much weight you need to shed, the next step is to calculate how many calories this represents. Lets say for example you currently weight 151 pounds (68.6 kilograms), and you decide you need to lose 20 pounds (9 kilograms). According to scientific assessment you have to burn off approximately 3,600 calories in order to lose one pound of fat weight. Therefore 20 pounds = 72,000 calories. For argument's sake lets also assume that you wish to lose this weight over a period of 4 months. That means that you will have to decrease your daily caloric intake by approximately 600 calories per day.

To maintain your weight at 151 pounds (68.6 Kg.) if you are an inactive person you would need to consume an average of 1963 calories per day. (If you were active your calorie expenditure profile would be calculated from an activity chart. Note must be taken that in order to even vaguely calculate calorie expenditure with some measure of accuracy it is necessary to determine not only the type of exercise and period of time, but also the person's weight).

So to recap; you wish to lose 20 pounds (9 Kg.) of fat weight over a period of four months. Your daily consumption would therefore need to be: 1,963 - 600 calories = 1,363 calories per day.

The next step in the process of formulating the diet would be to determine the quantities and types of foods whose caloric value equalled 1,363 calories per day. These values would be derived from calorie charts (see below). Some diets exclude certain foods from specific food groupings.

CALORIE CHART

	Calories	Protein	Fats	Carbohydrate
Apple 100gm				
USA source 1	81	0.3	0.5	21.1
USA source 2	58	0.2	0.6	14.5
Australia	35	0.2	0.2	9.0
Egg 100gm				
USA source 1	163	12.7	10.9	1.8
USA source 2	163	12.9	11.5	0.9
Australia	145	12.0	11.0	0.3

If you now examine the two examples that have been chosen, you will notice there are variances between the different sources, as well as differences between the various countries. Further, there is an even greater mathematical contradiction to this dietary approach, as Patrick Holford so clearly presents in his book *The Metabolic Guide*, the section titled *The Con Behind Calorie Counting*:

"*According to Dr Colgan, author of Your Personal Vitamin Profile, some of the athletes he works with burn off over 7,000 calories, but eat only 3,500 calories. By calorie theory, these athletes should have disappeared completely by now. An investigation by Dr Apfelbaum of people living in famine in Warsaw ghetto during the second world war show the same contradiction. With an average calorie intake of 700 - 800 calories per day, and a daily requirement of say 2,500 calories, a deficit of 1,241,000 calories would be built up over two years. The average body has 30 pounds of fat, representing 100,000 calories, to dispose of. Even if all this fat were lost, what happened to the remaining one million calories?*"

Patrick Holford goes on to say, *"the problems with calorie theory are not just mathematical ones."* The problems embrace the fact that the rigidity of diets ensure failure at some point for you must get hungry and break your diet. Calorie controlled diets are based on deprivation. If you are unable to enforce your diet through steely will-power you are doomed to break your diet. It must also be added that any attempt to restrict calorie intake will incline you to putting on fat weight. Hedi Lampert in her article titled *"How to Fool Your Fat Cells"* points out, *"Every time you go on a diet or deprive yourself of calories, your body becomes half as efficient at burning fat and twice as efficient at storing fat - and what's more, the effect is cumulative. In fact, dieting simply reinforces an ancient evolutionary survival tactic; the survival of the fattest."*[7]

The next stage in the process is to formulate the percentage ratios; in other words the relationship between the three main constituents of food, namely proteins, fats and carbohydrates. The ratios that are offered range between 15% - 30% for protein, 55% - 70% for carbohydrates and 10% - 30% for fats. In this area it is difficult to establish consensus. The debate also rages on as to whether you require 0.5 grams or 2 grams of protein per pound of body weight or whether in fact any of the percentage ranges have any relevance at all.

Well, you now have the basis to what is often regarded as a 'scientific' approach to dieting. At no point in this process can it be said that there was any consideration of the individuals varying needs. (This holds true for all dietary approaches.)

---

[7] From Style Magazine December/January 1994

In essence we are all vitally different - we each have our own unique fingerprint. Any form of diet must by definition preclude this consideration. We need to get back to the point where we can take pleasure in what we eat without the extremes of denial or obsession, and in so doing restore the body to its rightful place within an integrated whole. For if you truly eat to pleasure your body and not just your mind, you will eat what you need. The fulfilment of your natural needs ensures health, vitality and beauty. Your innate intelligence knows more than anyone else, what your varying needs are.

"Our natural physiological mechanisms are self-regulatory. Young babies, left to their own devices, choose all the foods they need to ensure healthy growth and development."[8]

If there is one thing that I have learnt over the many years of attempting to direct weight loss it is that when I started to connect intuitively the results far surpassed anything I ever achieved through dieting. In addition to the benefit of sustained weight loss there was the release of the mental and emotional anxiety that accompanies having to impose and maintain discipline. Eating once more became a pleasurable and rewarding experience.

Eating Intuitively

"Lurking just below the level of conscious thought is the world of intuition and the unfailing intelligence of the body. By becoming less preoccupied with conscious concepts and abstractions 'castles in the cortex' as

---

[8] *Overcoming Overeating:Conquer your Obsession with Food* by Jane R.Hirschmann and Carol H Munter published by Cedar.

some call them, we can reach into these deep wells wherein lie intuition, bodily intelligence and even the collective unconsciousness of the race."[9]

Intuition is a natural knowing - it is the summation of your mental, emotional, physical and spiritual wisdom. It is this deep *knowing*, this awareness that empowers you to move beyond the cyclical process of forever losing and gaining weight. This approach to losing weight and restoring vitality embodies the recognition that nutrition is an integrated approach; that what you think and feel has the power to affect the assimilation of nutrients. Similarly, what you eat has the power to affect your state of mind.

So far we have dealt with the various aspects of self-empowerment. This is the final phase, *eating for pleasure*. This is an easy, intuitive approach that embraces the awareness that your nutritional needs are dynamic; that they vary from day to day, moment to moment, and from individual to individual. As you go about your day what you mentally, emotionally, physically and spiritually experience, determines what you need to eat. Examples of this would be: if you ran up a flight of stairs on your way to the office, or if you were involved in a personal confrontation with someone, or simply, if a situation arose that was mentally vexing. All these situations would place different demands on your nutritional needs. Eating intuitively means eating what you need.

If you eat what you need you will not only be able to effortlessly lose weight and sustain this

---

[9] Article *The Instinctive Method: The Weider Instinctive Principle* by Franco Columbo in Muscle and Fitness July 1989

weight loss, but you will enjoy health, beauty and fulfilment.

There is no reason as you will see, why you can't enjoy eating and lose weight.

Before proceeding any further it is necessary to reiterate that **overweight is a choice.**. Overweight is something you create *"The habitual amount of fat you carry is not ordained by your genes. It is caused by what you eat and what you do.*[10] *We know now that neither the number of fat cells nor their size is genetically fixed."* It is also interesting to note that only about 5% of people that are overweight have metabolic problems. As Dr.Colgan points out the metabolic conditions of cortical or hypothalamic dysfunctions are generally the result of being overweight, rather than the cause of the condition.

Eating for Pleasure differs from dieting in as much as it is not prescriptive. Rather it concerns being in tune with your 'holistic' body. Intuition means being taught from within. It embodies a natural knowing. Only through the intuitive process of listening to your inner voice can you establish the internal rapport that is so vital to the process of losing weight. Rather than attempting to impose an approach from without that commits you to having to follow some rigid design, intuitive eating frees you from the polarities of either good or bad, healthy or unhealthy, success or failure. It is an inclusive rather than an exclusive process. It ensures that through an awareness of your mental, emotional, physical and spiritual needs that you make choices that benefit **You**.

---

[10] *Optimum Sports Nutrition* by Dr.Michael Colgan published by Colgan-Amino Research.

Intuitive eating is based on an awareness of your intrinsic needs and concerns eating what you need, when you need, rather than having to eat specific foods at prescribed times.

Your body is in essence comprised of subtle fields of vital energy. As such, whatever you think or feel has the inordinate power of affecting your body. If you are unhappy about having to control your eating or are forced to eat what you dislike, no matter that the food be regarded as 'healthy' this will manifest negatively.

"To a greater extent than we usually realize, our state of consciousness determines the way we transmute the levels of energy represented by foods."[11]

The power of the mind is that it has the capability to transmute either negatively, or positively the energy you derive from food. Intuitive eating is not based on any set of fixed principles or methods other than to acknowledge that it is necessary to honour all your various aspects. The more intuitive you are the more you will be able to effortlessly control your weight and direct your life.

Eating is driven either by *desire* (that of the mind), *response* (that of emotion), or of *need* (that of the body). As emotional responses are determined initially by what you think it is simpler to talk about mind and body rather than mind, emotions and body. Thus we either talk about eating from *need* or eating from *desire*. This does not necessarily mean that desire represents the negative and need the positive; rather, it implies that when we talk about eating from desire that it is indicative of a lack of harmony between mind and body.

---

[11] *Joy's Way* by Dr.W.Brugh Joy published by Tarcher, Inc.

The demand to eat comes from one of two sources. Either the mind sends the body a message that it desires food, or the body sends the mind a message that it is hungry. For most of us mortals we are governed by the former situation. Our bodies have been relegated to the sidelines in the interplay of mind and body - our minds run our bodies. The mind being all powerful overrides any feeling that issues from the body. Powerful gustatory images arouse the body into responding with consistent responses like; "Gee, I'm really ravenous", or, "I really could do with something to eat now". With these types of responses a whole mental video is turned on, replete with sensory images. Your taste buds are aroused and not only are you assaulted with evocative visual images but you are confronted by waves of feelings that assist in convincing you that you have to have that second helping of ice-cream, or whatever it is you so desire. The video takes over and you become obsessed with fulfilling your desire.

At no point in this drama did your body have any say. Your mental directives elicit the response they require from the body. Paradoxically, the body knows what it requires to function optimally but the mind being the more powerful in the relationship overrides the intelligence of the body. So in most situations, especially those related to eating, it is the body that is subservient to mind rather than an integration of mind and body. In some cases the mind is so powerful that even when our bodies give warning signs that something is seriously wrong, we still continue to abuse and pollute our bodies.

Pre-occupation with eating consumes much of our waking and even sleeping time. It is interesting to note that we generally only feel hunger when we think about eating. If we are distracted by something more interesting than food we forget our hunger. Think of a recent situation when you were totally involved in your work, your lover or some activity that you were completely immersed in. Did you think of food during this period? Were you faced with overwhelming pangs of hunger? In fact the more involved and greater your interest the less chance there is of being preoccupied by the desire to eat. This brings us to the point of acknowledging that our mental and emotional needs demand to be fulfilled. If we are unable to find the necessary fulfilment to these needs we substitute by eating.

The issue of eating inevitably gives rise to the following questions: What foods should you eat, and how much of these foods should you eat? These questions are only relevant if you ignore the vital relationship between mind and body. It is not so much an issue of what foods to eat or how much to eat, for this would lead us back into the realm of fixed and limiting concepts. Rather it is more important to re-establish balance between mind and body and in so doing *eat what you need*.

There is a natural consequence that takes place once all your parts are in harmony and that is, your need for those foods that are the very cause of overweight or illness disappears. In fact, you suddenly find that you are drawn to foods that are intrinsically more nutritious and beneficial to your body. The overwhelming desire to live on a daily intake of overprocessed and nutritionless food drops away and more often than not so too do your headaches, colds, allergies, and other ailments that are symptomatic of imbalance. For many symptoms of ill health are indicative of a body that is unable to cope with internal pollution. The digestion and metabolization of nutrients can't take place while your body is in chaos whether it be mind or food induced.

"There is no doubt that consciousness is affected by the quality and quantity of food."[12]

An intuitive approach to eating concerns being aware of your needs - being sensitive to what your body is telling you. In nature there are many examples of this principle at work. Have you ever noticed a creature in the wild to be overweight? I doubt whether you ever will for wild animals eat according to their needs. At an intuitive level they eat whenever they are hungry. At other times when they are ill they abstain from eating in order to allow their bodies to use all the available energy for the healing process. They do not eat according to some cerebrally determined dietary concept. They do not eat three meals a day at fixed times! Granted, that as human beings we generally go to work at certain fixed times and have to contend with mental and emotional intrusions that generally dominate our body's needs - but this does not prevent us from being receptive to the benefits of our innate intelligence. As Doris Grant and Jean Joice state in their book *Food Combining for Health:* *"Nature works continually to restore us to the ideal weight, stature, health, efficiency and everything else, when we remove the obstacles in the way of her remarkable healing power."*

The stated purpose of an intuitive approach to eating is to align your mind with your body and in so doing allow your body to participate and tell you what it needs. This means giving back some of the

---

[12] *Man and the Unknown* by Dr.Alexis Carrel (Nobel Prize Winner) published by Cath Art.

power to your body and becoming once more receptive to your body's judicious enunciations. When you are hungry, eat.

When your body indicates that it has had enough, stop eating. The body does not decide that in order for it to continue to function effectively (replace cells, pump the heart etc.) that it needs to eat excessively or that it should eat three regular meals a day or follow any particular diet. These are all constructs of the mind and social conditioning. Dr Hay, the founding father of food combining always advocated:

"Never eat anything of any kind at any time unless you feel really hungry.... You will get far more nourishment out of foods that are eaten when you are hungry than if these foods are eaten without proper hunger." [13]

Much of what intuitive eating is about is based on the fundamentals of a natural and common sense approach. Instead of structuring your meals around some 'abstract' timetable eat when you are hungry. Animals graze - they eat small amounts throughout the day. There is no reason why this will not work for you. Eating small meals throughout the day as you feel hungry speeds up your metabolism and ensures that your body receives a constant supply of energy. On the other hand eating three meals a day means that there will be periods during the day that your body is deprived of necessary nutrients. Any form of deprivation slows down your metabolism. This is the body's involuntary response - its protection against possible starvation. Slowing down your metabolism is fine if you want to gain weight. In

---

[13] *Food Combining for Health* by Doris Grant and Jean Joice published by Thorsons.

fact the Japanese Sumo wrestlers, some who weigh in excess of a few hundred pounds do just this. In order to put on as much weight as possible, they eat only a limited number of large meals. They also sleep after eating to slow the metabolism down even further. The other problem with eating only two or three meals a day is that by the time that you do sit down and eat you are so ravenous that you tend to overeat. But having said this, there may be times when your body demands only one, two or three meals a day. It all depends on your 'innate needs' - what feedback your body is giving you. It is important to appreciate that there are no rules! Rules are ordained by conventions - not by the needs of your holistic body.

If you eat what you need you will not put on weight. The body is only able to absorb approximately 20-30 grams of nutrient value at any one time. Anything that is in excess of this that is not excreted is stored as fat.

Structuring meals around some abstract timetable that aligns with your head rather than your needs is a sure way for putting on weight. The very notion of sitting down to prescribed meals at specific times can surely be only justified on the basis of social convention. This approach to eating denies the fact that you get hungry at different and irregular times of the day.

So, if you are not going to eat breakfast, lunch and supper at fixed times when should you eat?

When to Eat!

One of the fundamental principals to intuitive eating is that you eat whenever you are hungry. If that means six times or even ten times a day then that is how many times you dig in and eat. If you are hungry, then eat! Eat on demand. The more you are able to eat from hunger, the more you align with your innate need and the sooner you will lose excess weight. Overweight is only the result of im-balance, of not being in alignment. If you truly eat from need and not desire you will not gain weight. You may find this difficult to accept especially if you have spent years attempting to diet yourself back down to your natural bodyweight. It is very difficult to accept the notion of sanctioning eating on demand, for not only are we taught from young to restrain our appetite but we are also influenced by the social stigma of not being in control of our desires. What is vital is that you are able to re-establish the hunger/fulfilment link that you experienced as an infant when you were granted the right to suckle on your mothers breast whenever you were hungry. You need to reaffirm your right to eat whenever you are hungry.

Resistance to the notion of eating throughout the day is a reaction that is especially strong if you have dieted in the past. Dieting or self-denial are strongly linked to guilt. Obsessive behaviours like overeating are also strongly associated with feelings of guilt. The sequence of being driven to eat to fulfil a psychological need followed by self-flagellation for over-indulging is a sequence that alienates you from connecting eating with hunger.

The Denial Loop!

Any form of dieting reinforces denial. As you know, it is virtually impossible to endlessly perpetuate self-denial. Inevitably the next phase to denial is indul-

> *gence. You find that at some point your will-power fails you and you breakout and binge. With bingeing comes self-recrimination. Any form of emotional disharmony sets up a chain reaction. The denial/ obsession/ binge loop is once more activated.*

One of the ways that you can obviate this loop is to firstly become aware of this sequence. By beginning to re-connect the experience of eating with hunger you begin to ensure that you are fulfilling both your physiological as well as your psychological needs. How do you know that your impulse to eat is from need (physical demand), rather than from desire (mental demand)?

Need or Desire?

It is possible to *physically* distinguish between the *desire* and the *need* to eat. By physically locating where you feel the response you can identify whether it is being mentally or physically driven.

Generally the following pattern is observable: If your body requires nourishment then you feel this sensation somewhere in the abdominal area. On the other hand if it is being mentally stimulated (desire) then you will most probably locate the physical sensation somewhere in the region of the neck, mouth/ head area. I must caution you that there is always the exception. It is for you to discover where you feel these different sensations.

What to Eat!

Knowing when to eat involves also knowing *what to eat*. Knowing what to eat reaches into the very heart of intuitive eating. For, intuitive eating means that if you have a craving for chocolate that you recognize this need and that you eat chocolate without the attendant feelings of guilt. But, on the other hand, it also implies that addictions like living on a staple diet of crisps, chocolate and coke is indicative of imbalance - of being out of touch with your body. Eating with your mind and not listening to your body is certainly not intuitive eating. Yet, neither is denying what you mentally or emotionally feel. It is necessary to honour your mental, emotional, physical and spiritual needs. Intuitive eating is about balance - about integration rather than negation.

Intuitional eating embraces the understanding that all food serves a need - both nutritionally and psychologically. And, as your needs are not fixed you need to be able to respond to a wide variety of foods. There are no right or wrong foods! The only difference between one food type and another is its nutritional value. Food is not the cause of overweight, rather, being im-balanced is the cause of overweight - **Overeating Equals Overweight**.

If we briefly retrace our steps the first question you ask yourself when you start thinking about food is, "Am I really hungry?" If the answer is "yes", the next question must be, "What is it that I really feel like eating - what will satisfy my hunger?" These questions necessitate that you are sensitive to your body's needs. This includes eating not only those foods that are regarded as healthy, but also those so called 'forbidden' foods. The body's way of telling you what it needs may come to you in different ways. A craving for a certain food is telling you that you have a need for this food whether it be chocolate brownies, double-thick milk shakes or anything else for that matter.

Being sensitive means that as you begin to focus on what it is that you feel like eating, you visualize and imagine eating the food that has come up for you. There is no need for you to think about calories, fats, RDA'S or anything else. It is more important to get a sense of what it is your body needs. It is really not necessary to intellectualise this. Simply feel into the situation and discover what it is that you need to pay attention to. Start listening to those gentle suggestions that acquaint you with what your body needs.

At first you may find it difficult to establish what it is your body demands. One of the most simplest and most effective ways of dealing with this is by imagining those foods that you have a preference for. The more you go within and involve your body the easier this process will become. If it feels right, that is, the imagined experience of eating this food does not produce a negative sensation, then this food type is right for you. If not, think of something else you may like to eat. Run through this same process. Continue this until you find what will satisfy your need. I am sure you can readily recall a not so distant experience of feeling hungry and going into the kitchen. After munching your way through everything in the fridge you were still left feeling hungry. It was only when you were able to find that specific food that you had a hunger for that your need was fulfilled. In some instances this may be a mouthful that is required to meet your need. Hunger is not simply eating whatever comes your way or eating until you are full. Hunger is a distinct need that demands to be fulfilled in a specific way. This need is deeply connected to your mental, emotional, physical and spiritual needs. As such your hunger is associated with certain foods at certain times.

This brings us to the next point: if hunger is related to certain foods, then you no longer need to follow conventions like eating soup before your main meal, or eating dessert at the end of your meal. If your need is to eat dessert first then this is what you honour. Remember there are no rules to intuitive eating. If you have a need to have your coffee first, your desert second, and your main course last then this is what you do! Conventions were not ordained by nature!

If you truly eat according to your needs you are aligning with nature - and the consequence of this is that you will lose weight.

How Much to Eat!

The final piece to this jigsaw puzzle of nutrition concerns - *how much to eat*. Imagine the following scenario: you sit down to a meal and are served a plate of food. At what point in the meal do you stop eating? When is enough, enough? For many the point would be when they had cleaned their plate. For others, maybe even a second helping would be in order. The real issue that needs to be considered is not so much the matter of eating whatever you are served, but rather eating to fulfil a need. Once you have assuaged your hunger then this is the point at which you stop eating. Your body will soon send you a signal that it has had enough. One of the most effective ways of getting a reading from your body is to focus your attention on your abdomen area and register what you feel. Sensations that feel heavy and uncomfortable are indicative of having eaten more than you need. On the other hand, definite hunger signals indicate that you need to continue eating. When you eat be aware of the responses your body sends out. If what you eat causes bodily responses that are negative like indigestion, heartburn, discomfort, or any other similar response, honour this. One of the many benefits of becoming aware and attentive to your body is that your enjoyment of food increases.

Intuitive eating is the balance between all your needs. It is the balance between *knowing* and *sensing* what works best for you. The inclusion of all your needs, mental, physical, emotional and spiritual forms an integrated whole - for what you think feel, believe, or do, is inseparable and touches every aspect of your life.

"In the diseased system, the sensitivity to the body sensations is decreased and can lead to insensitivity to the body's needs, manifesting through improper diet, for example, which can create a negative feed back loop of more unbalanced energies. Each body that is disrupted or imbalanced also has a disruptive effect on the neighbour above it."[14]

Intuitive judgements are not the result of any logical sequences, but rather the instantaneous assessment of large masses of information. This includes both your conscious and unconscious aspects.

---

[14] *Hands of Light* by Barbara Ann Brennan published by Bantam Books.

Intuitive judgement is an integral part of your daily life. You use this natural form of knowing in your interaction with people and situations. It enables you to *feel* into the situation and make an assessment that would not normally be logically possible. Intuitive insight provides you with valuable information. In the case of being faced with danger intuition enables you to make snap decisions. There are many other impressive examples of your intuitive capabilities. Even the apparently simple situation of being able to jump from a height onto some designated spot is evidence of prescient intuitional perception. You may have never experienced this particular situation before, yet you are able to land exactly on target. Your intuitive ability to compute the height, the distance apart, speed of acceleration, trajectory and many other critical factors are mathe-matically complex to say the least. Nonetheless, your intuitive judgement immediately permits you to make the jump with great accuracy. To calculate the situation mathematically would be very complex to say the least.

Whether you are depending on your intuition to make snap judgements in critical situations or relying on this intelligence to eat correctly, intuition is able to provide you with access to a vast storehouse of knowledge and wisdom. John Davidson defines this aptly in his book *The Secret of the Creative Vacuum- Man and the Energy Dance:*

"So our instruments and devices are always simplifications of individual skills or functions which we ourselves already possess, in some degree....Only man, or a living creature, has an inward consciousness. Only in consciousness can we be simultaneously aware of so many factors in our environment. Con-

sciousness is the inward point of wholeness and integration, linking all our sensory and motor functions into one continuous experience. Consciousness tells us, through intuition within our mind, that the parts are integrated and connected into one whole."

Intuition can also be thought of as your inner guidance. By following your intuition you are following your natural flow of energy. This energy brings you insights and feelings that would not normally be available to you. As with any ability, intuitive judgement can be developed or allowed to atrophy depending on how much it is used and how much confidence you have in its results. It is necessary at this juncture to emphasis the point that it is not intuition that needs to be developed, for it is already fully developed but rather, it is your ability to allow this innate intelligence to reveal itself that requires development.

The first step in being able to open up to your intuitive wisdom is for you to begin honouring your intuition. Recognize that you have the capacity to be intuitive. This process involves learning to acknowledge that you can rely on your intuitive powers - that your intuition is capable of intelligent feedback. You can do this by beginning with everyday situations. Before answering the phone get a sense of who is on the other end, or, when you interact with others get a sense of whether they mean what they are saying. Feel what it is that lies behind their words. Also, begin taking cognisance of initial impressions when you first meet someone. Another exercise that is useful in developing intuitive awareness is to become aware of the different feelings that places have for you. When you enter a building or go out into the country become aware of the different energies that these places have. As you go about your day become impressionable to those places that you like and those that you do not. I'm sure if you momentarily reflect on this you will be able to recall the experience of feeling at ease or uncomfortable in certain locations. Once you gain assurance and open up to the benefits of intuition you will be encouraged to move onto more crucial issues.

There will be times when there will be an incongruity between what you think and what you intuitively feel. In these instances feel into the responses you are receiving. Get a sense of what lies beneath those thoughts that make you feel uncomfortable. It is really not necessary to intellectually obtrude into everything that you do, for intuition is a subtle state. Any attempt to control your responses will only cause you to miss what is being revealed.

The way to develop your intuitive awareness is to simply be sensitive to these subtle suggestions. It is not a process that you can direct. In fact the less you 'do', the more successful you will be. Intuition is of a delicate and tenuous nature. You cannot contain it. It is for this reason that no one can teach you how to be intuitive - being intuitive simply requires that you be sensitive and aware. If anything, being intuitive requires a surrendering of your ego, a stepping back, rather than an imposition of will. As you reveal the power of your mental, emotional, physical and spiritual bodies you will become increasingly more aligned. This alignment in itself will bring about an increased awareness of your intuitive powers.

With a bit of practice you will begin to sense the subtle difference between your intuitive responses and your mental intrusions. Once this starts happening you will be on an exciting journey of self-discovery. You may also find that what you think you feel to be your intuitive sense proves at times to be wrong. Do not let this deter you from exploring this wonderful capacity to benefit from this natural knowing. As you open to this exciting potential you will begin to experience a shift in the way in which you approach all situations. You will discover that the accuracy and pertinency of intuitive wisdom adds another dimension to the process of evaluation and response. This pertains to all situations, especially that of eating.

One of the consequences of gaining confidence in this subliminal wisdom is that you will find that you go with the flow. You will be less inclined to swim upstream. You will also realize that your actions are somehow more effective.

Lyall Watson in his book *Gifts of Unknown Things*, tells of an Indonesian fisherman who intuitively was able to sense and warn both the author and the islanders of an approaching tidal wave long before there were any visible signs of the impending disaster. The power and intelligence of intuition is unlimited. Like Lyall Watson's account there are many reports of 'primitive' societies like the Aboriginals of Australia, the South American Indians and the shamans of Mexico that are able to know things that are seemingly impossible to know beforehand "..... *There is a fund of knowledge, a different kind of information, common to all people everywhere ....inherent in the natural way of knowing is a sense of rightness that in this time of transition and indecision could serve us very well.*"[15]

---

[15] *Gifts of Unknown Things* by Lyall Watson published by Struik.

Intuition is a gift that modern man has scorned much to his detriment. Hopefully, as we reach forward into the future we will once again draw from this fount of inner wisdom.

Taking an intuitive approach to eating goes beyond the principals of scientific determinism. Intuitive eating certainly does not negate the advances of scientific research for intuition embraces all that we know. It is only through intuition that your individual and varying needs can be met. As you learn to trust in your intuitive responses and give back the power to your body you will discover that *'eating for pleasure'* is the key to losing weight and enjoying health and vitality.

Chapter Eight

A Passing Enjoinder

The process of living is an ever upward and onward journey of self-discovery. At times this journey will appear to be fraught with anguish and hardship. At other times it will be filled with joy. But whatever you may experience, you may be certain that these varied experiences are leading you forward. Every experience expands and ensures your personal growth and attainment.

Fat Equals Thin is by no means intended to represent the final word on self-empowerment. What is intended, is that in some meaningful way it provides you with the means to further your journey of self-discovery. The many paths that lead you to a deeper understanding of yourself can be likened to a spoked wheel. There are many spokes that lead from the rim to the hub. This is but one of those ways!

As you advance along the path of self-development you will bring to this process your own understanding. You will attract to you those influences and teachings that are necessary to your personal path of growth and realisation. In your quest leave no stone unturned. Encourage an openness to the way in which you view yourself and the world around you. Growth, whether it be spiritual, mental, emotional, or physical cannot take place in a climate of rigid acceptance.

As much as **Fat Equals Thin** is intended to assist you in losing weight, it is also intended to highlight the many other dimensions to your life. It is my deepest hope that in some way what you have touched on leads you to an awareness that your power lies within, not without. Through a process of opening up you can in your own unique way find spiritual, mental, emotional and physical fulfilment. As the Hermetic saying teaches, *"As above, so below"*. The omnipotence of All-That-Is is undeniably contained within your being. It only needs but be accepted to be revealed.

As you discover and develop your love of Self so this will flow to others around you. As you perceive the seed of magnificence within your being so you will extend this awareness to all of life. As you reach out and grasp your empowerment so your actions will uplift those around you.

May you fulfil your destiny as a unique and boundless being and in so doing find fulfilment, beauty and well-being.